RECLAIM
YOUR
HEALTH

David and Anne Frähm

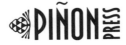

PIÑON PRESS

P.O. Box 35007, Colorado Springs, Colorado 80935

Reclaim Your Health
by David and Anne Frähm

Library of Congress Catalog Card Number: 94-24442
ISBN 08910-98690

Unless otherwise indicated, the illustrations in this book
are true to life and are included with the permission of
the persons involved. Any other illustrations are com-
posites of real situations, and resemblance to people
living or dead is coincidental.

This book is intended to introduce the reader to nutrition as an adjunct or alternative treatment for chronic
diseases, and to enable the reader to better understand,
assess, and decide whether nutrition and/or related therapies would be helpful and worth pursuing in his case.
This book is not meant to be prescriptive, nor should it
be used as a substitute for the advice of a qualified
health care professional. The author and publisher dis-
claim responsibility for any adverse effects resulting
from the information contained herein.

Frähm, David J.
    Reclaim your health : nutritional strategies for
conquering chronic ailments / David and Anne
Frähm.
        p.   cm.
    Includes biographical references (p.).
    ISBN 0-89109-869-0
    1. Diet in disease—Popular works.   2. Diet
therapy—Popular works.   3. Chronic diseases—
Diet therapy.   4. Nutrition.   I. Frähm, Anne E.
II. Title.
RM216.F82   1994
615.8'54—dc20   94-24442
                                          CIP

Printed in the United States of America

2 3 4 5 6 7 8 9 10 11 12 13 14 15 / 99 98 97 96 95

CONTENTS

Although both our names are on this book,
I (Dave) have been its primary guardian
as it has grown up and now left home.
I, therefore, feel the freedom, no, the privilege,
of dedicating this "offspring"
to my life's companion and cohort in adventure,
Anne Frähm.
For it has been her life
and her own story of health recovery
that have taken us down this path.

ACKNOWLEDGMENTS

Traci Mullins, editor and friend: Thank you for your vision for our books and your labors at giving them birth.

Mike Leming, publicist, friend, and another visionary for our message: Thank you for helping us deliver it to the public.

(Two behind-the-scenes servants, underpaid for all their labors, yet not underappreciated by those for whom they labor.)

Charlie Fox, friend, fellow health advocate, and yet another who has seen into the future concerning the impact of our mesaage: Thank you for providing a platform.

All the people who shared their stories with us, only a fraction of which form the contents of this book: Thank you for your willingness to open your lives to others.

HOW TO USE THIS BOOK

This is a book of stories, not blueprints. They are meant as examples of what has worked for others, not exact prescriptions to be followed word for word by you, the reader. What is contained in these pages should not be used as a substitute for your personal interaction with a qualified health care professional who can thoroughly assess your unique biochemistry and design a program tailor-made to your own specific needs. If you need help locating such professionals in your area that use nutrition and related non-toxic therapies, we do keep a list. See the resource section at the end of this book for more details.

Although these stories are not meant to be prescriptive, they are nonetheless illustrative of the principles of nutritional healing—(1) cleaning out and detoxifying the body, and (2) rebuilding its various systems, particularly the immune system, through a diet based largely upon plant foods and dietary supplements. We would all be well advised to take heed to such principles.

Should you like to contact any of the individuals whose stories make up the pages of this book, that may very well be possible. Most have given me the freedom to give out their phone number to anyone who would ask. Call us here at *Health*Quarters (719)593-8694 and we'll see if we can link you up.

BRINGING NUTRITION INTO THE MAINSTREAM

It all began with a tiny lump. Anne found it while she was doing one of those things women are supposed to do with their breasts every now and then. It's great to get good news from a doctor, especially when a mammogram is in his hand. But when he says everything is okay, and it really isn't—when you go away happy and relieved, only to learn later that what was considered a benign cyst has spread legions of rebellious cells throughout the body to form new outposts of life-threatening disease—then that's not so good, that's not so happy. In fact, that's hell. And for us, that's how it all began.

So what do you do when you find out that your body is being eaten alive from the inside out by an onslaught of renegade cells referred to as cancer? You do what the doctor says, right? You do the surgery, and if it means allowing some part of your body to be amputated, so be it, because you want to survive. And you do the radiation. Letting a technician burn parts of you with laser beams, permanently damaging some of your tissue or organs, is part of the game. And chemotherapy? Of course! Even though it, too, damages your organs, impairs your immune system, and otherwise devastates your whole body. And what if your cancer finally becomes resistant to all attempts to beat it down? Well, then you try a bone marrow transplant that leaves you secluded in an isolation room in some remote hospital for fifty-two days, throwing up your guts and teetering on the brink of death. That's all the right stuff to do, isn't it?

But what if even that is not enough? What if in the end, after all that you've gone through, endured, and tried under your doctor's care, cancer is still in your system and growing back rapidly? What then?

That's where we found ourselves several years ago. "Go home. Eat, drink, and be merry. Squeeze all the life you can out of your days, because we think you don't have many left." That's what the medical types were telling Anne, at least those we had personal contact with. From their point of view we'd exhausted the options. Nothing else to do. Nothing else to try. The curtains were closing in on my wife. Soon it would be time for her to bow out. At thirty-six, she probably wouldn't see thirty-seven. Time to buy a plot and arrange for the organ music.

That's when it happened. A watershed experience. Something so vitally important that it changed our lives, facilitated the return of health and vigor to my wife's body, and redirected our contribution to this world. In short, we met a nutritionist! Okay, okay—perhaps not as exciting as winning the lottery or going out to lunch with a movie star, but for us, it was revolutionary.

At first I was skeptical of what this so-called "nutritionist" might be trying to "sell" us. Would I find feathers in her office—as in "quack"? People say that it's part of human nature to get set in our ways, becoming resistant to new ideas, new truths, and change. I could certainly identify with that. My "German-Iowan" heritage served to keep me firmly rooted in the familiar. This idea of fighting cancer with food seemed just too odd and suspicious for me to embrace with open arms.

Another, and perhaps even more passionately felt reason for my initial apprehension stemmed from my philosophy of life. You see, both Anne and I are committed followers of Christ. Christianity is the path along which we've chosen to make sense of the world, creation, and life. I was more than a little concerned that the whole idea of natural healing through nutrition and related nontoxic therapies was going to be contrary to my worldview—more of an "Eastern religion—New Age voodoo" kind of thing than truth with a biblical basis. I had visions of chanting mantras over bowls of broccoli, or being urged to become my own god.

As it turned out, this unusual new acquaintance held our same views on life. It was her strong conviction that God had entrusted our bodies to us as gifts and expected us to take care of them. For her, "taking care" included learning how to feed ourselves properly, something she had learned firsthand as she had fought her own battle with tumorous disease.

Just five weeks after launching ourselves on a very strict program of detoxification and nutritional rebuilding through a radically changed diet, accompanied by a huge regimen of dietary supplements, Anne's cancer was gone (see the full story in *A Cancer Battle Plan*, Piñon Press, 1992). Vanished. *Finis.*

Looking back, it's obvious to us that the conventional therapies did help to initially reduce the cancer load in Anne's body. However, it's just as obvious that without "nutritional-metabolic" therapies and related lifestyle changes Anne would no doubt be dead. Unfortunately, no one we knew in the medical community at that time was even hinting to us that there were other options, other opportunities, other avenues to explore outside mainstream or so-called "conventional" medicine. We were left to find them on our own. But as we did, it was like going from black and white to color.

AMERICANS WANT OPTIONS

We are not alone in having found that there is more to health care than the narrow picture represented by drugs and surgery. According to a recent study conducted by Dr. David Eisenberg of Boston's Beth Israel Hospital and published in the *New England Journal of Medicine* there is growing acceptance by health-care consumers of "alternative" practitioners and their methods.[1] Fully one-third of all Americans are seeking help outside the flow of mainstream medicine, and spending nearly fourteen billion dollars a year to do so. With insurance companies slow to recognize the validity of many of these alternative therapies, consumers are left paying three-quarters of this bill out of their pockets.

So, what are so many of us looking for, and willing to sacrifice so much money toward, when we venture outside the boundaries of the mainstream? Perhaps most would identify with the words of this mother as she stands in the doorway watching one of her young sons being treated for asthma by a trusted acupuncturist:

> "I do go to the doctor when they're very sick. Just because I go here doesn't mean I've abandoned Western medicine. But I've found that when you go to a regular doctor, they'll listen to you, then give you a prescription for the symptoms—and not deal with the underlying problems. Here they try to get more at the root of the problem."[2]

More and more people are going to alternative therapists for one reason, and one reason only. Better results. We're not fools. We're not out to throw our hard-earned cash to the wind. We want to feel better. And if current conventional medicine doesn't work, we want the freedom to try something else.

Health care in the U.S., just like everything else, is a consumer-oriented, results-driven business. Put up, or shut up. Competition is the name of the game. If something's not working, we don't want to be pressured to stick with it just because the practitioner has a wall full of medical degrees and belongs to the politically powerful and domineering American Medical Association (AMA). To acquiesce, of course, would be politically correct. However, more and more Americans are becoming politically incorrect regarding their health. One might call them "medically incorrect."

Don't misunderstand. This book is not anti-doctor or anti-modern medicine. It would be foolish to say that mainstream medicine does not have a significant role to play in the health of our society. In some situations, the U.S. has the best medical care in the entire universe. It's just that drugs, surgery, and radiation aren't the answer to *every* question concerning the complexity of human health. The scope of health and healing extends far beyond the collective training and expertise of the family doctor, internist, surgeon, and oncologist—as should our options for treatment. As health-care consumers, we need—in fact, we demand—information and access to all our options. We want alternatives, and the freedom to choose. Unfortunately, the power brokers in mainstream medicine don't always feel like the customer should have that right.

In 1963, for instance, the American Medical Association (AMA)—the trade and lobbying group for mainstream medical professionals—came up with what they thought was a great idea. They formed what they called a "Committee on Quackery." I guess at that point in their history they figured that they had a corner on everything there was to know about the human body and its health. And since they'd become such a political powerhouse in the U.S., they set about to squelch any philosophy of health care that differed from their own. In many ways their actions resembled those of Russia's Stalin who, after deciding he alone knew what was best for Russians, killed off all who disagreed. The AMA's main target was chiropractors. Of course they didn't want to kill them, just put them out of business. Chiropractic science and its practitioners were labeled "unscientific." The AMA passed a snooty decree that it was unethical for a physician to associate with such as these.

Well, the whole thing backfired on them. In 1976 a chiropractor took the AMA to court for antitrust violations. The trial lasted eleven years, resulting in a ruling by a federal judge that the AMA was guilty of conspiracy and could no longer attempt to prevent members from associating with these fellow professionals with a differing viewpoint and specialty. With that, the AMA wandered away to lick its wounds, disbanded their Committee on Quackery, and no longer had an official position on what is termed "alternative medicine." Today, chiropractic is considered by many professionals as part of the mainstream of American medicine, even covered by "physician-driven" insurance companies. As some astute observer once said, "New truth is at first coolly ignored, then vehemently opposed, and finally warmly embraced."

Back at the acupuncturist's office the treatment has been completed. A week later the woman's son is breathing freely. She's thankful that she's found a practitioner who has really helped him. "I can just look at him and tell he's doing much better." Mission accomplished. His asthma is under control. And this without toxic drugs and their side effects.

Is Nutrition Just Another Option?

Under the heading of "alternative" health-care therapies, a number could be listed, each adding its unique contribution to the big picture of the administration of health in this country. They are represented by such diverse practitioners as chiropractors, homeopaths, herbalists, acupuncturists, naturopaths, massage therapists, colonic therapists, reflexologists, and nutritionists, among others. We've already referred to acupuncture and chiropractic, each of which has made significant strides toward greater recognition and acceptance within the widening scope of health care. Others—like homeopaths and naturopaths, who practice natural means to stimulate the body's own healing mechanisms—are gaining ground with the public, if not with mainstream physicians. But perhaps no other field deserves more of our attention as a country than does the field of nutrition, referred to by some as biological medicine.

Every year 700,000 Americans die of heart attacks, 520,000 die of cancer, and another 162,000 bow out due to strokes. Are you aware that the current statistic is one out of every three Americans will develop cancer at some point in their lives? That number promises to become one in every two by the year 2000. Currently, 50 percent of all Americans will develop heart disease at some point in their lives. Cancer, heart attacks, and strokes—the top three killers of Americans—are related primarily to what we feed our bodies. Pick up any newspaper or magazine these days and you're bound to find an article or two acknowledging this truth. "Diet and lifestyle," observes John A. McDougall, M.D., "are the causes of most of the deaths and disabilities that people suffer in the United States today."[3] And the outlook in many other Western countries is almost as bleak.

Granted, we will all die of something sooner or later, but why not make it later? Life is precious. It is a gift from God to be treasured and used wisely. There are things to do, places to go, people to see. Unfortunately, we're eating ourselves into early graves. Heart attacks and strokes, for instance, are the leading cause of death and disability in men forty to forty-five years of age. And cancer is no longer considered the sole property of the aged. According to the American Cancer Society's *Cancer Statistics* published in the late 1970s, more people are dying from cancer at an early age than at any other time in recorded history.[4]

Then there are those bothersome ailments—things like allergies and arthritis. Although typically not life threatening, they can still make life miserable. They eat away our enjoyment and impair our productivity. The evidence is clear that many maladies of the human machine are very much related to what we put into our "tanks." (For more detailed information, see our book *Healthy Habits*, Piñon Press, 1993.) We just can't ignore the truth. What we feed our bodies can and does have either a positive or a negative impact on our health.

The practice of nutrition is not just an option, not just an alternative in the field of health care. It is a must. A mandate. Nutrition is a science that needs to be considered foundational to all other health-care practices. The health of the human body is built on what it is fed. Not only does nutrition help to prevent disease, but it can also help to reverse it.

So What *Is* Nutrition?

For the purposes of this book good nutrition is defined as anything consumed by the individual that helps to deliver to his or her cells the kinds of nutrients needed to keep those cells functioning properly and at peak performance. Obviously this includes the kinds and quality of food we eat. But it also includes the quality of the air we breath (oxygen is the single most important nutrient for human health), the quality of the water we drink, and even the sunlight we expose our skin to. (Again, you may want to look into *Healthy Habits*.)

To this list we must also add the category of dietary supplements. These include herbs, vitamins and minerals, amino acids, enzymes, etc. They are added to a diet to help compensate for imbalances or deficiencies and, in some cases, to help fight certain disease processes. For instance, vitamins A, C, E, and the mineral "selenium" actually have anti-tumor effects. (We've said more about this in *A Cancer Battle Plan*.)

A third and final category rounds out the definition of what is meant in this book by the practice of nutrition. You've no doubt heard the popular saying, "You are what you eat." That's only partially correct. The whole truth is, "You are what you absorb." A vital part of the nutritional process involves ensuring that the body is in the necessary condition to fully utilize what is put into it. You could put the best food and supplements in your stomach; you could breath clean air and drink purified water; you could do all that's well and good to do—yet still be in terrible health, if your body is unable to use what you've given it. It's interesting to note that 40 percent of all cancer patients die *not* from the disease, but from malnutrition—the inability to absorb nutrients.

Such an unfavorable condition as malabsorption arises when a person develops what is referred to as a toxic "overload." The organs and individual cells can become so overwhelmed by the onslaught of pollutants taken in with food, air, water, and medications that the body eventually becomes unable to flush them clean effectively. Essential to the effectiveness of the nutritional approach to illness and disease is the purging out of these contaminates, a process called "detoxification." Without cleansing, your cells are unable to fully absorb what they need to maintain proper functioning.

Nutrition, then, has to do with food, air, water, sunshine, vitamins, minerals, other supplements, and the body's ability to absorb and use all of these. You are about to be introduced to a host of people from around the U.S. (and the world) who have used nutritional therapies to fight back against various negative health conditions, either in themselves, their children, or their clients. In some cases, nutritional therapies alone were employed; in others, nutrition was incorporated into a broader agenda. Some of these people have completely reversed their symptoms. Others are still in process, but making good progress. All acknowledge the vital role that nutritional therapies play in their own battle plans.

My hope for you, the reader, is that you will come away from your involvement with these people with a firm conviction that you, too, can make significant improvements in your own health by what you put into your mouth.

QUOTES

"When I was a medical school student . . . the study of nutrition was very sketchy; even today most doctors are painfully ignorant of the real advances in nutritional science. I began to suspect the close relationship between health and proper eating habits when, early in my career as an overworked young doctor, my own health broke down. I have always been a man of great curiosity and as I investigated deeply the chemistry of food along new lines, I came to the conclusion that I, personally, must give up the use of drugs and henceforth rely solely on food as my medicine. It wasn't long until (after repeated verified results) I discarded drugs in treating my patients."

—Henry G. Bieler, M.D.
FOOD IS YOUR BEST MEDICINE

"As a doctor, I knew about the importance of nutrition, but, like most physicians, had not taken the time to look at the real state of the art in nutrition research. Years ago, when the University Hospital swallowed me along with the other frightened medical students, we had too much on our minds to think about healthy eating. . . . We were terrified of drowning in the long hours of demanding, detailed work. Nutrition, preventive medicine, and health in general never figured into our thinking. With junk food stuffed into our pockets and plenty of black coffee and cigarettes, we were determined only to survive."

—Neal D. Barnard, M.D.
THE POWER OF YOUR PLATE

"If you are a patient, you may know more about nutrition than your doctor. Nutritional information is beginning to sweep the world like a prairie fire because it does make sense. People are becoming well as a result. They are looking for a doctor who understands the nutritional concept. There are practically none. If you are a doctor and if you will catch up with the demands of the public, your future will be far more assured than ever before. You will again achieve that image of respect once accorded you in yesteryear. You will truly satisfy the

requirements of your Oath of Hippocrates. Best of all, you will get, and keep, most of your patients well. Your services will be in great demand. I know, because it happened to me."
　　　　　　　　　　　　　　　　　　—Alan H. Nittler, M.D.
　　　　　　　　　　　　　　　　　　A NEW BREED OF DOCTOR

"Many patients have been restored to health through the practiced application of biological medicine after all the conventional treatments have failed. Biological medicine and naturopathic methods of treatment will come to the fore more and more as the successful alternative to conventional therapy; and for the afflicted, who tried in vain conventional therapy, they present the only choice. The philosophy of biological medicine is not in opposition to conventional medicine; it rather widens, deepens and complements it."
　　　　　　　　　　　　　　　　　　—Lars-Erik Essen, M.D.
　　　　　　AS QUOTED IN THERE IS A CURE FOR ARTHRITIS
　　　　　　　　　　　　　BY PAAVO AIROLA, N.D.

"Perhaps the idea of caring for your own health or do-it-yourself health measures are incompatible with the American way of thinking. Americans have been educated to believe that you have to 'go to your doctor' for any health advice; that studying and reading about health and practicing sound hygienic and dietetic health principles is the pastime of crackpots and 'health nuts.' No doubt, this attitude is to a great part responsible for the fact that the average American is so ignorant regarding his own health and the proper means of maintaining it. We are health-conscious, yes—but only superficially. We are confused and ignorant as to what are the correct means, nutritionally and otherwise, to assure optimum health."
　　　　　　　　　　　　　　　　　　—Paavo O. Airola, N.D.
　　　　　　　　　　　　THERE IS A CURE FOR ARTHRITIS

"Doctors who use alternative methods, such as nutritional therapy, are not careless and are not renegades or irresponsible. They are probably the most conservative and careful of physi-

cians because they don't want to do anything that can harm their patients. I'm the same way."

—Priscilla Slagle, M.D.
AS QUOTED IN *THE NUTRITION REPORTER*

"Many people already are aware that doctors are woefully ignorant in nutrition. Only about one-third of the nation's 125 medical schools require students to take courses in nutrition, and most of those courses are very brief. This is a shocking statistic, considering that 6 of the 10 leading causes of death are directly related to diet.

"Seven years ago, the National Academy of Sciences recommended that medical schools greatly expand their nutritional education, yet the number of medical schools requiring nutrition courses of any significant length is about the same as it was in 1980.

"Why is there such resistance to change? According to Dr. Marion Nestle, Chairwoman of the Department of Nutrition at New York University, the bottom line is money. Preventive health services such as nutritional counseling by doctors, are not reimbursable by the government or insurance agencies. Another factor is that new doctors need to make a lot of money to pay off the heavy expenses of medical school, so they gravitate to specialties that pay well.

"There are problems on other levels, as well. Because doctors aren't trained in nutrition, there aren't many physicians who are qualified to teach the subject—a self-perpetuating problem. Also, there is a limit to the number of courses that will fit into the curriculum, and entrenched doctors on the curriculum committees don't want to take any time away from their own specialties. According to one expert, the old guard is so firmly entrenched, improvement in the nutritional education of doctors cannot be instigated at the medical school level, but must be nationally mandated."

PREVENTION IN ACTION NEWSLETTER
American Preventive Medical Association (APMA)
Dr. Julian Whitaker, M.D., President

NOTES
1. David M. Eisenberg, M.D., et al., "Unconventional Medicine in the United States: Prevalence, Costs, and Patterns of Use," *New England Journal of Medicine*, No. 328, January 1993, pages 246-252.
2. Rhoda Archuleta, as quoted by Warren Epstein, "Americans Check Out Health Care Alternatives," *Colorado Springs Gazette Telegraph*, November 28, 1993.
3. John A. McDougall, *McDougall's Medicine: A Challenging Second Opinion* (Piscataway, NJ: New Century Publishers, 1985), page 286.
4. American Cancer Society, *Cancer Statistics* (New York, NY: Professional Education Publication, 1979).

2

NUTRITION AND AIDS

Introduction to AIDS and HIV

Certain death. That's what many of us have come to believe is the fate of anyone who contracts the disease called AIDS. AIDS is an acronym for "acquired immune deficiency syndrome," an impairment of the body's ability to fight disease. A person who has it is left without protection, vulnerable to illness that a healthy immune system might otherwise overcome. A certain form of pneumonia and a rare skin cancer are two of the more common opportunistic diseases associated with the AIDS condition.

So does AIDS, itself, actually attack and wound the immune system? No! AIDS doesn't cause a non-functioning immune system. AIDS is the result of an already non-functioning immune system.

As the name says, AIDS is an "acquired syndrome." It's a condition, not a cause—the end result of something else's impact on the body. That "something else" is called the human immunodeficiency virus (HIV). Today's headlines warn that HIV can lead to the AIDS condition. Great precautions have been undertaken throughout society to avoid the mingling of blood or body fluids between individuals, the most common routes of transmitting the virus.

HIV and AIDS are scary. A lot of people have died. There are some, however, who have successfully managed to fight back through nutrition and related natural therapies. They are showing a way through the valley of the shadow of death.

ROGER COCHRAN, M.D.

The horrors of Vietnam left deep wounds in the lives of many people who served there. For some, the scars were visible. Day in and day out, helicopters delivered the maimed and mutilated GI's from the battlefront to blood-stained operating tables where gallant doctors struggled mightily to patch and repair what the enemy had tried to destroy. Fifty-eight thousand didn't make it. Countless others came home with broken bodies, evidence that they'd been to hell and back.

And *what of* those doctors that labored in pools of blood hour after hour? Did they, too, share in the wounds of the battlefield? How could they not! The stress and horror of trying to salvage body parts on fellow human beings and piece them back together again penetrated and victimized even the most well armored of hearts and minds.

"A lot of good men couldn't handle the stress and went to pieces in Vietnam," acknowledges Bob Smith, M.D. He ought to know, he was there. So was Roger Cochran, friend and fellow graduate of UCLA Medical Center. Roger was one of those doctors who cracked. "The constant pressure of it all got to him, and he turned to drugs," says Smith. "A lot of doctors did. As well as medics. And nurses. And GI's. The miracle is that we all didn't."

Cochran was lucky. He got himself rehabilitated and was issued an honorable discharge. After Saigon fell and he and Smith eventually arrived back in the States, they lost touch with each other. That was until one day, years later, when Roger showed up in the doorway of Smith's office.

"I always did say that you were the best doctor I knew," said Cochran to his long-lost buddy. "The best diagnostician. The best with patients. And that's why I've come to you. . . . I'm depending on you. I'm depending on you to find a way to save my life!"

Roger Cochran, M.D., had AIDS.

The story of Roger's recovery through the help of his friend Bob Smith, has been documented in fascinating detail in a book by Bob Own, Ph.D., simply titled *Roger's Recovery from AIDS*.

It's a story of two men and their rebirthing process. For one, a rebirth from "sure" death to life. For the other, a rebirth into a new understanding of how the body works to heal itself and the role of a physician to assist it.

Step by step in his journey toward new understanding, Dr. Smith was made aware of the vital role of the body's own immune system in health and healing. The work of others often prodded him forward. For instance, the thoughts of Paavo Airola, Naturopathic Doctor, on arthritis. Smith stumbled across a book Airola had written called *There Is a Cure for Arthritis*:

> While drugs and injections may relieve pain and modify symptoms, they do not go to the bottom of the problem, they do not eliminate the underlying causes, nor do they correct the systemic disturbances. What is even worse, these conventional remedies, being suppressive in nature and having undesirable toxic side effects, interfere with the normal bodily process, and actually inhibit restoration and healing efforts of the body. Eventually, they cause more damage than good, and lead to a complete invalidism. . . . It must be emphatically stated that drugs do not possess curative powers. The cure is always brought about by the body itself, and the most that a wise doctor can ever do is assist the body's own healing forces.[1]

"In that moment of discovery," recalls Smith, "I knew as well as I knew my own name that the healing philosophy Airola was espousing was not earmarked for arthritis alone. Airola was speaking of basic principles that applied to disease in general. All kinds of disease."

Armed with a new understanding of his role as facilitator of the body's powers to heal itself, Dr. Smith went about the process of creating an environment in which Roger Cochran's immune system could work toward restoring itself. The hope was that if his immune system could be regenerated, it could go to bat against the high levels of HIV in his bloodstream. In other words, instead of treating the disease, Dr. Smith sought to build up the body's fighting forces.

How the HIV had invaded Roger in the first place was uncertain. He wasn't homosexual, so that was ruled out. He had been around a lot of blood in Vietnam. He'd also been addicted to illegal drugs during those years. Perhaps the virus had been injected via a contaminated needle. But that was long before anyone had even heard of HIV and AIDS. Perhaps his post-war medical practice in San Francisco was the key. It had brought him in contact with many AIDS patients.

But how he'd gotten the virus wasn't nearly as important as what he'd do about it. Up until now, much of his lifestyle and diet had served to further weaken his immune system—opening the door for full-blown AIDS development. Although he'd kicked the illegal drugs, he'd since become hooked on the prescription stuff. He'd also been treated for a tumor in his abdomen with radiation and chemotherapy (both are extremely hard on the immune system), after which he never fully regained his weight or strength. On top of this was his insatiable addiction to sugar and caffeine. It was not unusual for him to consume twelve to fifteen cups of coffee a day, with half a dozen teaspoons of sugar in each, besides the usual Cokes with lunch and dinner. Radiation, drugs, sugar, caffeine—all enemies of the immune system. For years Roger had subjected his immune forces to heavy attack.

The environment Smith eventually created to help his good friend rebuild his immune power, piecing it together as he went, addressed internal *and* external needs. In order to clean out the buildup of toxic wastes in Roger's body from years of poor diet and drug abuse, a fast was instituted. Only fresh juices were to be taken. Externally, Roger was placed in a stress-free environment where the worries and cares of life would be temporarily prohibited from sending negative signals and bad chemistry to the rest of his body.

Three weeks into the fast—he stayed with it for a total of five—Roger's health began to show improvement. Minute, at first, but improvement nonetheless. Steadily, his blood profile improved and his color returned. It was an almost unbearable detoxifying process that was nearly interrupted on several occasions by Roger's desperate pleas for medication, coffee, anything that would help deal with the pain. Smith stood fast, although doubts certainly haunted him. He was, after all, trained within the hallowed halls of conventional medicine. Who'd ever heard of fasting as a health-promoting form of therapy? For that matter, who'd ever heard of denying a patient pain medication?!

"It was very plain to me that the medical profession, including myself, had not actually had anything to do with Roger's return to health. Roger's body, when provided the opportunity, had done the job itself! Doctors and drugs had not been needed. X-rays and hospitals, with their huge facilities and staffs had not been utilized. Yet prior to Roger's dramatic return to health, he had been drained by the medical profession. They had accepted his money, sliced him open with scalpels, poked him full of holes into which they had poured drugs and from which they had drained blood. They had practiced their deadly game of drugging upon him until it became clear that nothing worked. They had failed. Yet they were unwilling to accept biological alternatives as viable options. Instead, they had made their full and final decision: They declared him 'untouchable,' tacked a 'terminal' label on him, and shoved him out into the cold. From that point on, Roger's only future was the grave.

"As a medical man myself, I knew that all physicians were not so crass. I knew that there were thousands of compassionate and concerned doctors who were pouring out their energies to keep their patients alive and well. But it now seemed obvious to me that AIDS, per se, was much more than just another disease or epidemic. It was an institution. A carefully designed institution. And that behind the 'AIDS scare' a huge and powerful money machine was calling the shots and controlling the entire pharmaceutical and health-care industry."

Roger's Recovery from AIDS is a "must read, must give copies to others" type of book. Its value lies not only in its help and hope for those battling AIDS, but for all of us who need to learn better ways and means of taking care of our immune systems. (See "Further Reading" list on page 36.)

KAREN WHITE

It's been a hard life for Karen White. I could tell that the lady on the other end of the phone had been "toughened" by her experiences. She's had cancer three times, undergone a hysterectomy, been kicked out of the Navy, tried to kill herself on an eight-month cocaine binge, and wound up sitting in jail. To top it all off, now she has AIDS.

"While in the Navy, I was originally diagnosed with Hodgkin's disease," she explains. "Following that, I had cancer in my thyroid and my uterus. No big deal. I wasn't going to let something so simple as a little cancer get me down."

Her Uncle Sam, however, had other ideas. After her bout with uterine cancer, she was issued a medical discharge and told to go find a cure. Along the way, a new set of doctors discovered that not only did she have the Big C, but the Big A as well. "Back when the hysterectomy had been done to remove my diseased uterus, I had to have blood transfusions. That's when I got contaminated blood."

Discovering that she had more to worry about than she'd thought, Karen's emotions hit the skids. "That's when I went on the cocaine binge. I was working as a bartender. People tipped me with drugs. I thought my life wasn't going to amount to anything with this disease, so I basically tried to commit suicide. I ended up getting myself arrested."

But Karen's a tough person. Picking herself up by her bootstraps, she's managed to make a go of her life after all. Today she sees herself as sort of a "spokesmodel" for AIDS. An unenviable role to say the least, yet one that makes her feel good about making a contribution to her world.

"I make my number available so I can talk to others about AIDS. In fact, that's where I was last night, giving an AIDS talk to a bunch of parolees. That's a real easy job. Usually they ask me how to keep from getting the HIV virus. I tell 'em, masturbate."

That, of course, is her way of promoting abstinence. She doesn't mince words. AIDS isn't a "words-mincing" disease.

As for her own battle plan, Karen has included many strategies. Nutrition, however, has been front and center. Has it helped? "Oh, yes, definitely. Pneumonia is one of the big killers of people with AIDS. I'd had it four times before getting in with a naturopathic doctor. She put me on a special diet and a regimen of vitamins and minerals—things like A, C, E, zinc, herbs, and cod liver oil—to help rebuild my immune system. Over the last several years I've had the sniffles only once, and I've avoided the flu altogether. When I realized that the drugs they give to AIDS patients weren't going to rebuild my immune system, I stopped taking them. Even the AZT, the drug commonly prescribed to fight the HIV virus."

What do her previous doctors think about what she's doing?

"They're behind me in whatever I do," she says with a bit of a chuckle. "They can't be much against it, since I'm not following their program but I'm still getting better."

Karen White's plans are not just to survive AIDS, but to conquer. Judging from the fight that's in this warrior, AIDS hasn't got a chance. "And once I get myself cured of all this," she says with a great deal of confidence, "I'm going back to the Navy and make them take me back."

BILL SALAZAR

"Well, Bill, you're gonna die. But before you do, you're gonna go blind. And before you go blind, you're gonna. . . ."

Okay. Okay. He'd gotten the point. Bill Salazar sat in a doctor's office listening to him pronounce his death sentence. "That guy was the most depressing, sad person I'd ever met in my entire life," he recalls. "In fact, my wife named him 'doctor death.'"

Being HIV-positive, of course, is certainly no walk in the park. Bill had picked up the virus through homosexual contact years before, and now he faces a sizable enemy, one that has cut down many before him. However, HIV doesn't necessarily lead to AIDS and death. As Bill points out, "Nutritionists claim that less than 50 percent of the people who are HIV-positive develop AIDS." A fact that gives him hope.

According to what he's learned, the HIV virus hides in the

immune system. If a person lives or eats in such a way as to decrease immune power, the virus will be able to multiply and spread. However, a health-promoting lifestyle and diet will keep the immune system strong, increasing the potential of keeping the virus in check.

A growing number of medical professionals are pointing toward the rebuilding of the immune power through nutrition and related natural therapies as the key to winning the battle against AIDS.

In his book *Healing AIDS Naturally*, Laurence Badgley, M.D., recounts the stories of eight men who cured themselves of AIDS through a combination of natural therapies to rebuild immune power, focused heavily upon nutrition. He makes the following observations:

> It should be emphasized that the stories you read here [in *Healing AIDS Naturally*] are not the only ones. Many more exist. The eight men described have regained their health . . . in the face of astounding obstacles. Up to the present time, the official credo has been that AIDS is fatal and follows a progressive downhill course. These men courageously took their medical care into their own hands at a time when all the institutional support groups, doctors, and other "authorities" presented a completely dismal picture of the AIDS disease process. Nor did they practice their natural therapies in secret. They practiced them in full view of their friends and peers, who often openly denigrated their undertakings. "Oh, so you are going to go and eat a carrot for your AIDS!," was one retort. These survivors accomplished their successes while the witnesses to their recoveries often discounted what they saw. According to some of these survivors, many of the witnesses to the events . . . were themselves ill with AIDS. The astounding thing is not that these survivors got better. The astounding thing is that many of the witnesses . . . chose not to similarly pursue their own course of natural therapies! The way we choose to view the real world shapes our own reality. Many of these witnesses are now dead. I think that this phenomenon makes a powerful statement

about the society we live in, the knowledge base that we live by, and the lemminglike behavior of humans in general to unconsciously follow their medical doctors wherever they wish to take them.[2]

Bill Salazar is seeing a medical doctor to monitor his condition, but that's not all he's doing. "The doctor I have now has been monitoring HIV-positive patients who have remained symptom free for over fifteen years. They are that way because they've taken it upon themselves to care for their immune systems through nutrition and lifestyle changes. I plan to do the same.

"The thing is," Bill continues, "most people in the HIV boat have the attitude, 'Hey, I've got the virus, I'm going to die anyway, so why not live it up. Nothing I can do will matter, anyhow.' So they sign their death certificate with their ensuing lifestyle."

What the medical world has to offer does little to challenge such a fatalistic attitude. According to what Bill has discovered, AZT can eventually do more harm than good. It ultimately destroys bone marrow and causes severe anemia. In addition, this potent drug causes liver, kidney, and neurological damage and destroys intestinal cells, resulting in wasting disease. Other drugs are being developed that may prove less toxic, but Bill remains wary.

Bill's concerns about the damaging effects of AZT and other drugs on AIDS patients are shared by a growing number of medical professionals. Findings being published in the *New England Journal of Medicine* indicate that while AZT does seem to delay the onset of full-blown AIDS, once it does develop, the early users of the drug tend to be sicker and have more AIDS-related problems. In the end, AIDS is more quickly fatal for AZT users.[3]

Alan Cantwell, Jr., M.D., observes that "more than a decade after the introduction of the AIDS virus into the US population, the results of recommended treatments for HIV infection remain disastrous for the patient. . . . Obviously, something more is desperately needed other than the official FDA-approved drug therapy for AIDS."[4] He suggests what we've already discussed: Evidence is mounting that certain dietary measures and nontoxic therapies can help fight HIV and AIDS.

Ironically, even though the physician currently monitoring Bill has patients who are using nutrition against their virus with good success, he has nonetheless suggested to Bill that he start the drugs.

"Well, first of all it will take your body some time to get used to the drugs, probably at least six weeks. You'll get real sick— vomiting, no appetite. You'll bleed from your eyes and fingernails. Your fingertips will turn purple. And you'll have pain and difficulty urinating, accompanied by severe diarrhea."

"Are you nuts! You want me to take something that is obviously toxic and will compromise my immune system!?"

"Well, when your body gets used to the drug, the T-cells that are such an important part of your immune system will go up."

"Okay, then what? Can I expect a number of years of good life if I take these drugs?"

"Well, actually you'll probably have about six good months. Then the virus will adapt to the drugs and start to multiply again. After that, you'll probably develop full-blown AIDS."

It never has been completely clear to Bill why his doctor would recommend such a course of treatment. Maybe for legal reasons, he was required to. Who knows? Whatever the reason, Bill has flatly refused. And just like this doctor's other patients, he's seeing good success with nutritional therapies recommended by a local nutritionist.

"Because of my nutritionist's program of detoxification (fasting and enemas) and rebuilding (raw, organic fruits and vegetables with dietary supplements), my T-cell count went from 800 to 1289 in just a month and a half. Helper cells went from 320 to 350. A flu that was going around, which my wife got and suffered with for ten days, lasted in me just twenty-four hours. At my nutritionist's advice I did a megadose of vitamin C every hour, plus a coffee enema every two and a half hours. No medications, no aspirin, nothing. In fact, a cancer I'd had on the roof of my mouth cleared up as a result of her program."

It's obvious to Bill that maintaining a strong immune system through nutritional therapies is an important key to an effective HIV battle plan. He'd had a previous doctor, however, who refused

him as a patient when he found out he was using nutrition.
"He said, 'You're looking great! Your weight's good. Your color's good. Your blood pressure's good. What have you been doing?'

"When I told him I was using nutrition, he threw a fit.
"'Don't you know that those people are quacks, charlatans?! They're just out to take your money. Sure, you're going to look great! Sure, you're going to feel great! But the bottom line is, you're going to die anyway!'

"There are some doctors out there like that guy who love to play God," observes Bill. "'If we can't help you,' they say, 'no one can. You're gonna die.' They tell you that their way is the only way, or that AZT is the thing to do, even though it's a death sentence to everyone who takes it and the FDA is considering taking it off the market. That already happened once, when AZT was used primarily for cancer patients. Problem was, it was killing everybody. Too dangerous. So now they're giving it to HIV and AIDS patients?"

Bill's mention of AZT and "death sentence" in the same breath is understandable given the hard facts. A five-year study in Great Britain showed that "individuals who tested HIV antibody positive but were asymptomatic died more quickly and in greater numbers if they were given AZT."[5]

Fortunately, the doctor Bill sees now, even though he has suggested the AZT, is willing to monitor his condition even though he has opted for the nutritional route. "I keep seeing him for tests and blood work," says Bill. "Every time he suggests drugs, I just say no."

QUOTES
"There are many more case histories of HIV positive patients . . . who are conquering their diseases by reversing the downward slide of their immune systems. No longer need AIDS be the number-one public health issue facing the United States, and the world, today. AIDS can be stopped!"
—Morton Walker, Doctor of Podiatric Medicine
TOWNSEND LETTER FOR DOCTORS

"There is increasing evidence that malnutrition is a major cause of immune deficiency, morbidity, and mortality in AIDS patients. Anecdotal reports indicate that correction of nutrient deficiencies results is a significant improvement in clinical status, fewer opportunistic infections, and longer survival. Nutrients currently recommended for AIDS patients include vitamin C, vitamin E, zinc, vitamin B_6, vitamin B_{12}, folic acid, and coenzyme Q_{10}."

—Alan R. Gaby, M.D.
TOWNSEND LETTER FOR DOCTORS

"AIDS is a chronically manageable infection, and will prove to be a curable disease, it's just a matter of time. . . . I have developed what I call, the five point empowerment program for the treatment of HIV disease. Now note, I did not say the cure of HIV, but the treatment. . . .

1. Stress reduction

2. Dietary changes . . . largely vegetarian

3. Supplemental nutrients . . . vitamins C, A, E, B, and the major minerals, coenzyme Q_{10}.

4. Drugs . . . do play a role, but I think a minor one . . .

5. 'Nutrition for the Mind' . . . visualizations, affirmations, forgiveness exercises, massage classes, learning deep breathing, taking a stick to a tree and just beating out their internal feelings, public service for other causes, etc."

—Joan C. Priestly, M.D.
JOURNAL OF ORTHOMOLECULAR MEDICINE

FURTHER READING

AIDS Control Diet by Mark Konlee (West Allis, WI: Keep Hope Alive, 1993, 5th edition), P.O. Box 27041, West Allis, WI 53227.

Healing AIDS Naturally by Laurence E. Badgley, M.D. (Forest City, CA: Human Energy Press, 5th printing, 1990).

Roger's Recovery from Aids by Bob Owen, Ph.D. (Cannon Beach, OR: DAVAR, 1987), P.O. Box 1100, Cannon Beach, OR 97110.

NOTES

1. Paavo O. Airola, N.D., *There Is a Cure for Arthritis* (West Nyack, NY: Parker Publishing Company, Inc., 1968), page 34.
2. Laurence Badgley, M.D., *Healing AIDS Naturally* (Foster City, CA: Human Energy Press, 1987), pages 40, 54-55.
3. As reported in "Study Finds AZT Can't Lengthen Life," *Townsend Letter for Doctors*, May 1992, page 334, by UPI.
4. As quoted by Mark Konlee, *AIDS Control Diet* (West Allis, WI: Keep Hope Alive, 1993, 5th edition), under "Comments" section.
5. As reported by Jule Klotter, "Lies and Misdirection," *Townsend Letter for Doctors*, May 1994, page 416 (book review of *Dirty Medicine* by Martin J. Walker).

3

NUTRITION AND ALLERGIES

INTRODUCTION TO ALLERGIES

Typically, we think of allergies related to inhalants—the dusts, pollens, danders, and molds that populate our lives and pester our airways. In many people's minds the word *allergy* conjures up images of someone suffering through the hay fever season with a box of tissues in one hand and a package of antihistamines in the other.

But an entirely different realm of allergy must be considered—in fact, two realms that play very significant roles in the health of the human body. The first is *food allergies*, the subject addressed in this chapter. The second is *chemical allergies*, addressed in the chapter "Nutrition and Environmental Illness" (see pages 148-169).

Theron G. Randolph, M.D., is a pioneer in the field of treating people who are suffering from food allergies. He's helped thousands. In his book *An Alternative Approach to Allergies*, he makes the following observations about those whom he's treated:

The majority of these patients have been helped significantly, often after conventional methods of treatment had failed. Sometimes patients have come to me with a single well-defined ailment. Typically, however, patients have been polysymptomatic, that is, they have had a long history of many problems, physical and mental, which had left them in a general state of misery. The more symptoms they accumulated, the less their doctors have believed their complaints.

Usually, neither patients nor their physicians have suspected food allergy as the root of their problem. This is because most food allergy, by its very nature, is masked and hidden. It is hidden from the patient, hidden from his or her family, and hidden from the medical profession in general. It is said that often the solution to a difficult problem is right in front of your nose, but you cannot see it. In the case of food allergy, the source of the problem is literally in front of you, in the form of some commonly eaten substance which is bringing on and perpetuating chronic symptoms.[1]

What follows are stories of people who have suffered through the frustrations of not knowing what was wrong with them or their children, finally discovering that the answers were to be found in the foods they were eating.

A.W. PICKEL, III

Mr. Pickel had a problem. He hated his own guts. You see, right about the time he turned thirty he began to experience terrible abdominal pains after every meal. They'd send him hunched in agony toward the nearest couch.

"I was really struggling," he recalls. "After every meal I'd have to lie down because I was having such severe cramping. Once I could finally get to my feet, I'd have to B-line it to the bathroom with the 'runs.' Diarrhea, you know."

As one might guess, eating out was always a real adventure in timing for the Pickel family. Invariably, the pains would hit him right in the middle of the ride home. Gripping the steering wheel like a man holding on for his life, he'd try to keep the contents of his colon from exploding.

Finally, things got to the point where something had to be done.

A. W. needed an answer to what was happening to him. A full battery of tests was scheduled, including a barium enema. Time to get to the bottom of this dilemma. No pun intended, of course.

"First, they gave me this stuff like Pop Rocks candy and said, 'Swallow, but don't belch.' Immediately a huge gas bubble started growing in my stomach. Then they took some of the same stuff and stuck it up my other end, and they told me, 'Don't fart.' So there I was, gas bubbles the size of both my thighs growing in my groin, and they tell me, 'Strip.' Well, okay. And then they said, 'Stand here,' and they brought this cold metal thing up against my body. They said, 'Hold your breath.' That wasn't all I was holding!"

Before it was all over, A. W. had undergone a full-scale reconnaissance of every nook and cranny of his intestinal track and related vital organs. The doctors report: Nothing wrong. No intestinal problems, no ulcers, no trouble with the prostate . . . nothing.

Sometimes good news can be as frustrating as bad. Your mind buzzes: What do you mean nothing's wrong?! Come over to my house for dinner tonight, and while I'm lying there on the couch in pain, tell me once again that nothing's wrong. But the doctor had spoken. Tests don't lie. The $1,000 he'd forked over had been money down the proverbial toilet.

One day while talking to a friend, A. W. happened to mention his health problems. "Sounds to me like we're talking about a lactose intolerance," his friend observed. "Maybe dairy products are your problem."

A. W. Pickel had always been big on dairy. His main diet in high school had been a thoughtfully selected menu of Hostess Ding Dongs, accompanied by the mild bouquet of "moo juice" chasers. Later in his married life, wife Diane would greet him at the door of their urban cottage after a hard day at the "salt mine," holding in her loving hands a plate full of melt-in-your-mouth chocolate chip cookies and a big glass of something white and cow-like to wash them down.

A lactose intolerance, huh? Well, it was worth investigating. In fact, anything that might be even remotely helpful was worth a shot at this point. Eating was getting to be a very frustrating experience.

That very day, A. W. made it a point to avoid all dairy products at lunch. Gone was his customary glass of milk. To his immense surprise and utter delight, gone too were his customary "after meal" pains.

Could it be? Was it possible? Were dairy products truly the culprit behind his months of agony and frustration? Naw, that would be too simple. Wouldn't it?

To test his hypothesis, a glass of milk was added that night to his evening cuisine. Within fifteen minutes his guts were in knots. But this time the pain was mixed with rejoicing. The mystery had been unraveled. Eating could once again be an enjoyable experience without the promise of a painful aftermath. All he had to do was avoid dairy products.

Sometimes the simplicity behind our physical ailments is profound. According to nutritionally aware health-care professionals, most people are simply not equipped to digest cow's milk. In fact, cow's milk is the worst offender for the development of allergies in humans. Could it be that God intended only calves to drink cow's milk? Many health-care professionals think so.

ROGER AND JAN CROSS

The Cross family has lately had a lot to bear. Not long ago, Jan's mother came for a visit. She'd been suffering for months with excruciating muscle spasms in her back.

"Mom's doctor had done a complete bone scan and found nothing," says Jan. "He figured it was arthritis and told her to take ibuprofen whenever it hurt." (Some doctors' idea of treating an illness.)

Problem was, it hurt a lot and it hurt all the time, like someone had stuck her in the back with a knife. She was sending acetaminophen, ibuprofen, and aspirin down the hatch like they were going out of style. Five pills at a pop weren't touching the pain. Mom was frustrated, her kids were frustrated, and her kid's kids were frustrated. Life in the Cross household had become very tense.

One morning Jan remembered that a friend had recommended a local chiropractor who was also a nutritionist.

"I got his number and called. Bless his heart, he came in on his day off to see my mother. He spent a couple of hours with her, doing muscle response testing to identify what sort of foods she was allergic to. He took her off a bunch of stuff, including dairy products, sugar, and caffeine. That was a Friday. By Tuesday the muscle spasms had disappeared."

Wow! Talk about getting results. Jan and Roger decided to bring him their own list of health problems. Roger had been plagued with an inner-ear problem for years. His previous doctors, of course, treated it with antibiotics. These had not helped. In fact, by the time he found this new guy, Roger had developed a ferocious yeast infection. Antibiotics, after all, kill off not only bad bacteria but also the good organisms, which would normally keep the naturally occurring yeast in check. Without the "yeast police" around, it can go on a destructive rampage throughout the body, destroying tissue and zapping energy. (See chapter 6, "Nutrition and Candida.") If you can imagine a 100-watt light bulb getting only 50 watts of power, that was Roger. Not quite the image of death warmed over, but close—very close.

And the best way to deal with this beast? Starve it. Avoid eating foods that feed it. These included all yeast products—breads, pastries, and processed foods of various kinds. It's amazing how much of what we normally eat contains yeast. Roger also had to avoid food products containing vinegar or mold. This included catsup, mustard, salad dressings, mushrooms, and cheese. Finally, anything with sugar was also removed from his diet. That's a biggie. Almost all processed foods you can buy in the grocery store contain some form of sugar. Plus the natural sugars in fruits need to be avoided, at least at first. Additional dietary changes were made to help with the clogged ear. Dairy products, in particular—the notorious producers of mucus and congestion—were to be avoided.

In a matter of months, Roger had beaten back the yeast infection. His inner ear problem had also improved about 50 percent. The hope is that it will continue to get better as he keeps working on his health through nutritional means.

As for Jan, her health complaints stemmed from the fact that she was struggling through "the change"—menopause. Pain had haunted her every move for the last five or six years.

"I wish I had been aware of nutrition and made some dietary

changes years ago," she confesses. "I'm convinced it wouldn't have been so rough on me physically if I had. Going through menopause was really ripping up my body."

Indeed, she was a mess. Her whole body would ache and be sore to the touch. She had pain in her upper abdomen, mid to lower back, right shoulder and arm, neck, and legs. Often she'd wake up at night with terrible cramps in her feet, and would have to get up and soak them in hot water to relax the muscles. Mornings greeted her with leg pains.

"It was this awful experience going through menopause that finally made me open to issues of health and nutrition," she admits.

Their newfound nutritional consultant put Jan on a diet of greens, salads, vegetables, rice, beans, and fruits. He recommended that she lay off the sugar, dairy products, and caffeine. Through muscle response testing, he also discovered that she was extremely allergic to gluten, the stuff in wheat. That meant no breads, pastries, or pastas made with wheat.

As a result of the changes she made in her diet, Jan's health dramatically improved. "When I eat right I don't have all those horrible aches. Plus, I've lost my hot flashes. But when I eat wrong, the pains all come back. Last week, for instance, I took cinnamon twists over to friends who were moving. It was hard for me not to sit down and have a couple with them. I hadn't eaten what I shouldn't for a long time. That night I was in misery once again. It'll probably take my body a couple years to build up to the point where I can indulge myself in some of those foods I'm now to stay away from."

Jan and Roger Cross are working toward a vegetarian diet. They still eat meat, maybe three times a week, but are moving toward a more plant-centered menu.

"We've come to really enjoy this diet," says Jan. "Personally, I've been awakened to the taste of food in a way I've never experienced before. I love fruits and salads. I used to just tolerate them. I'd drown my greens in blue cheese dressing. I didn't actually taste anything but the dressing. Now I eat salads all the time, and if I put anything on them at all, it's just a little canola oil and maybe a little bit of salt for taste."

Their two daughters have also jumped on the wagon, particularly their high schooler.

"Last year she'd come home from school and sleep for two hours on the sofa every day," Jan recalls. "We had her see our nutritionist, and he took her off all the foods she was allergic to—gluten, dairy, and night-shade vegetables (specifically tomatoes). She was also to avoid sugar. As a result, she no longer comes home tired and in need of sleep. Her energy level is amazing. It's a total change. She's a basketball player, and it's even changed her game. She used to kind of just lumber down the court because she didn't have the energy. That's changed. It's obvious that dietary changes have really helped her performance. Even her attitude and temperament is affected. The other day she said, 'Mom, I'm a nicer person now.' She's right. She's just not as grouchy as she used to be. Before, she was so tired and out of it. And it was all because she ate the wrong kinds of foods."

You can tell that the Cross family is thankful for what they've discovered about better health through nutrition. But at the same time, Jan has this warning: "After eating one way for years, don't expect nutritional changes to improve your health overnight. You won't see overall, long-term change until after you've been at it for a while. I still have some sore places in my abdomen, like they've been bruised for a long time because they were abused by what I put in my stomach. It's going to take some time to heal."

Healing their health, that's what the Cross family has been doing. It does take time and effort. Good health does not come automatically. But the results are well worth the investment.

AMY WILLIAMS AND SON

Amy Williams knows the world of medicine from the inside out. As a nurse, she's seen firsthand the good that modern medical treatment can render in certain situations. She's also seen its ineffectiveness. Her own story is a case in point.

"I'd been having sinus infections for eight years. It all started when my son was born. First I'd get one a year. Then two. Then three."

Every time, she'd take antibiotics. They'd help for a while, but sooner or later, infection would come roaring back. In an effort to change the course of things once and for all, Amy tried surgery. "The two sinus surgeries I had didn't help at all. Getting my tonsils out did help briefly, but then I began getting stuffed up and infected again."

It finally got to the point where Amy developed the mother of all sinus infections. It lasted for two years and cost her the job at the hospital.

"I got to a point where I couldn't even get out of bed, much less take care of my family. I was on the strongest antibiotic available, but it wasn't touching my fever. I went in and told my boss I had to quit."

Prednisone is a steroid, a "wonder drug" doctors often prescribe to mask symptoms caused by incurable conditions. To take it means throwing in the towel to a disease—"You can stay, but I don't want my immune system to know you're here." It stifles immune system response to foreign invaders it should otherwise respond to. Although the body is fooled into thinking that nothing's wrong, it's like putting a Band-Aid over skin cancer. You might not be able to see it or feel it, but it's there and getting worse.

"That was the last thing my doctor had to offer me—Prednisone, every day for the rest of my life. As a nurse, I knew it would devastate my immune system and eventually destroy my adrenal glands, but I was looking for anything that would help. I tried it for four days and was getting psychotic. That stuff can really play havoc with your head. I knew that wasn't the route I wanted to take."

She also consulted with an allergy doctor. He told her to get central air conditioning, remove all the carpeting in the house, get rid of the pets, and dust the place three times a day. Was that the way to go? She wasn't sure.

In every story there is a turning point. For Amy it came when she went to see a chiropractor who did muscle response testing for food allergies.

"I found out which foods I was allergic to, began detoxifying my body, ate only organically grown foods, and took vitamin and mineral supplements. It's been over a year since I began eating and living this way, and I'm feeling so much better, I can hardly believe it!"

Amy's son has also responded with enthusiasm to his mother's newfound formula for better health. Since the age of two he'd been a sickly kid. On and off antibiotics. Terrible ear infections. Horrible stomachaches at night that would wake him up crying.

"My son twice had operations on both ears to put in tubes to help with infections. At two-and-a-half he had his tonsils out. He was still sick, sick, sick all the time. He barely made it through second grade, having missed so much school. He was always on antibiotics, fighting off infections, falling asleep in class. And until he was about eight, he was very overweight."

When Amy saw what dietary changes had done for her, she immediately put her son on the same regime. "We took him off dairy, sugar, wheat, and all processed and refined foods. In the first month he lost fifteen excess pounds. He had felt so bad that he wouldn't even go out to play. He'd come home from school and just collapse. All that has changed with his new diet. And he doesn't cheat. I grind fresh grains every morning for breakfast. And I send all his food with him to school and when he goes on overnights with friends. Beans, rice, carrots, celery, apples, sometimes a few corn chips. He used to get teased, but he's getting strong and taller than the rest of his friends. He tells the other kids, 'Hey, maybe if you eat like I do you'll grow up someday, too.'"

Amy the housebound invalid has gone back to being Amy the nurse, hired again in her old job. She's still fighting off some yeast overgrowth brought on by the heavy use of antibiotics. (See chapter 6 for more information.) Otherwise, she's doing fantastic and has added her voice to the growing chorus singing the praises of nutritional therapies for better health.

"I see people every day who are sick and have no hope of ever getting better. They're often struggling with things that could be helped through nutrition. But if you say anything to them about changing their diet, they're not into it. They just want the doctor to give them drugs and make them better. Trouble is, drugs won't make you better."

KIM ELMORE AND KIDS

Imagine, if you can, a life governed by hourly medications, as many as six treatments a day on a special machine, and several emergency hospitalizations a year, all done in an attempt to keep you doing the simplest of things—breathing.

Such was the fate of two children in the Elmore family, both under the age of three. Each had been diagnosed by pulmonary pediatricians as asthmatic. Each had been prescribed mounds of medications and special machines that blew soothing steam into their faces to help them breathe.

"The kids would be pretty wired each day on the medications," recalls their mother Kim. "And at night I'd have to wake them up periodically to give them breathing treatments on the machine, or clap them on the back to help get fluid off their lungs. If they ever had an asthmatic attack, they'd be taking about seventy breaths a minute. That's very serious. Off to the hospital we'd go."

Each had been in and out of hospitals more often than their parents wished to recount, and much more often than their insurance company wished to repay.

At one point early on, child number three, a daughter, was hospitalized with respiratory distress. Spending a week inside a special breathing tent, the medication alone cost $3500. Before this crisis had arisen, the Elmores had changed insurance companies. This second company tagged her illness as a "preexistent condition" because her brother had the same illness. That was the excuse given for not paying up.

There wasn't much life for Mom outside the confines of the house and taking care of the two sick kids. The treatments on the steam machine had only short-lived results. Within thirty minutes the good effect would be all but gone, and the tightness and congestion would begin to set in once again. The list of medications the kids required would have kept a small country well supplied. Kim kept a chart, broken down by the hours of the day, indicating who needed what and when. It became her taskmaster; she, its slave.

"It was all very time consuming and exhausting. On top of that, the kids weren't getting any better," Kim recalls. "It would have been worth it had they been making progress, but they weren't."

Finally, after two years of this sort of tortuous lifestyle, a friend recommended to Kim that she take the kids to see the doctors at the Environmental Health Center in Dallas, Texas. Just six weeks after starting a new program of therapy, the kids no longer needed any kind of special respiratory help. Wow! In fact, they've been free of asthmatic symptoms for over eighteen months since.

So what was the magical medicine that the good doctors at the Center dispensed? "Instead of treating our kids for asthma," says Kim, "they considered their asthmatic condition the final result of other things that were happening to them. In other words, instead of treating the symptoms, they looked for the causes. They found that both kids were allergic to several different kinds of foods, and several different airborne allergens."

The whole of the therapy consists of an allergy shot twice a week, plus a changed diet. In relative terms, simple. No more charts and hourly medications. No more around the clock visits with the steam machine. No more frustrations that things just aren't getting better. What a difference! And all because someone, a group of trained professionals, made it their practice to search out the reasons behind reactions—the causes behind the symptoms.

The Elmore's doctor at the Environmental Health Center added these instructions to their program, "When you feed your kids fruits and vegetables, make sure they're organically grown. In other words, keep the pesticides out of their systems. Their bodies are so sensitive when they're young, they'd feel a greater impact than an adult would. And definitely stay away from plain tap water for drinking. You don't want all those chemicals and pollutants in their bodies."

How does Kim feel now about all they went through with their kids to get to this point?

"It's pretty frustrating," she says as she reflects back. "We're out thousands and thousands of dollars that insurance didn't cover. And all the traditional doctors kept telling us, 'Yes, your children do probably have allergies, but they're too young to be diagnosed.' We found out that this simply wasn't true."

What would she say to other parents of children who display asthmatic symptoms?

"Well, some children truly are asthmatic. They were born with deficient lungs. But it's worth investigating to see if the asthma is allergy induced. If so, it can be controlled. My heart goes out to all those kids who have been misdiagnosed, like my own kids were, and continue to suffer needlessly."

JOHNNY BLUE STAR

Johnny Blue Star. Radio host and producer, screen writer and playwright. A man of many talents. A man who likes to communicate. There was a time in Johnny's life, however, when simply taking a good breath was the goal, much less communicating.

"As a child I had a lot of bronchial problems, difficulty breathing, constant mucus. Allergies were part of my life. I knew I was allergic to a lot of different things—pollen, animal hair, chocolate. . . . The combination of allergies and the inability to breathe made my childhood less than fun.

"I had the standard American diet. Meat, potatoes, and lots of dairy products. I remember drinking milk and waiting for the rush of power the TV commercials promised. I could never get that feeling from milk, but I assumed it was there because I really bought into the idea that milk was indeed good for me."

By the time Johnny had entered his late teens and early twenties, his allergy and breathing problems seemed to all but fade away. He remembers nothing specific that he'd done to help himself. Maybe it was just that his immune system had somehow been bolstered. For whatever reason, he remained symptom free for a time.

"When I moved to Manhattan, New York, however, all those problems came rushing back into my life. I developed a cough that simply wouldn't give up its hold on me. My doctor diagnosed me as asthmatic. My breathing finally became so labored and my coughing so bad, that the only way I could control it long enough to speak to others was by using codeine. Yet even that was becoming increasingly ineffective."

At the same time, Johnny had developed eczema on his hands—itching, swelling, peeling skin. The doctor gave him some salve to suppress the symptoms, but warned him he'd be dealing with it for the rest of his life.

In the midst of these health problems, a job change landed Johnny in New Orleans. The humidity of the deep south made his attempts at breathing even more labored and troubled.

"When I got off the plane, I was immediately struck with air panic, the feeling that there was no air and that I was drowning. Compounding this panic was the fact that I hadn't slept well for months, the mucus in my system made me cough so much. I really felt like I was going to die. I thought I would have a heart attack right then and there because I was breathing so hard. It was a frightening experience, to say the least. And it was obvious that my ability to communicate with others was decreasing because of my inability to breathe."

One day as he was riding through town on a trolley, Johnny spotted a health food store. It caught his eye because of the name, Helen Keller's Health Food Store. At first he was reluctant to pay it a visit because of the association with blindness. Eventually he wandered in.

"What's wrong with you?" was the greeting he received. "You look terrible!" The woman had addressed him in a thick, German accent.

"Asthma," he sputtered.

"Asthma? That's nothing! Last year I cured a fourteen-year-old girl of leukemia!"

Johnny looked her in the eye and thought, *This is a nut!*

Her name was Helen Keller, obviously not *the* Helen Keller. She was a chiropractor by profession and owner of the health food store. She started showing Johnny around, in particular she wanted him to see an article about the girl she'd helped beat leukemia.

"Part of her program involved juice fasting with carrot juice," Johnny recalls. "I thought that was one of the most absurd things I'd ever heard. I went home thinking to myself again, *This person truly is a nut.*"

That night, as had become his pattern, Johnny didn't sleep well. But this time it wasn't just because the mucus in his system was making him cough and wheeze. The phrase that had been

planted in his head that day kept playing itself over and over—
"Asthma? That's nothing!"

The next morning, Johnny returned to the health food store.
Desperate times call for desperate measures, even if it did mean
teaming up with a "nut."

"I don't know who you are or what you're into," he huffed
toward Mrs. Keller, "but I'll do anything you say if you can just
make me better."

That morning Helen Keller began to unfold for Johnny Blue-
star the wisdom behind what she called a mucus-less diet. She put
him on a liquid fast using vegetable broth and carrot juice. A variety of herbs were also to be taken.

"Within three days I could feel the mucus drying up in my
bronchial tubes," recalls Johnny. "I was beginning to be able to
breathe freely again. It was amazing. I hadn't thought it possible.
I'd been led to believe that my problem with asthma was beyond
help."

Johnny discovered that his symptoms were set off by a variety of foods and environmental pollutants—allergies. "I found that
if I walked into a place with a lot of carpet, I would begin coughing, and I'd feel a reaction on my skin. I also discovered that dairy
products and sugar really set me off."

At the same time that he was working on his new diet, he
discovered in a book by Adele Davis that asthma and eczema
are sometimes linked. PABA was supposed to help—part of the
B-complex vitamins. He took a dose and within twenty-four hours
his supposedly incurable eczema had disappeared.

Later on in his road to health, Johnny developed a rash all over
his body. He looked into every possible cure, consulting with seven
or eight different doctors. In the end, an herbalist friend suggested
that he add some acidophilus to his diet. Acidophilus is the friendly
bacteria which prevails in the intestine and keeps the harmful bacteria in check. It does a host of different things that are good and
important for health, including producing B vitamins in the body
and helping clear up skin problems.

"I took the acidophilus and within an hour my rash was completely gone."

After all his experiences, what does Johnny Blue Star think about health care in the U.S.?

"Just like there's a law at abortion clinics to tell the client about all of her options, I think every medical doctor should be bound by law to explain natural means toward healing with all of their clients."

QUOTES

"Food allergy is the most commonly undiagnosed medical condition in the United States today."

—James Braly, M.D.
DR. BRALY'S FOOD ALLERGY AND NUTRITION REVOLUTION

"Many diseases are due to the body's reaction to ingested foods, chemicals, and pollutants. The body is trying to tell the owner that something is wrong."

—Lendon H. Smith, M.D.
DR. LENDON SMITH'S LOW-STRESS DIET

"Most medical treatment for allergies is not curative but is aimed at reducing symptoms. Ideally, we want to correct and heal the body so that we become less congested and less allergic. Before even thinking about medical investigation and treatment, it is wise to do what we can ourselves first. . . . Changing our diet itself can aid in preventing and treating all kinds of allergies, especially those to foods, which are very common. Often, just eliminating 'reactive' foods from our diet can reduce symptoms of other allergies."

—Elson M. Haas, M.D.
STAYING HEALTHY WITH NUTRITION

FURTHER READING

An Alternative Approach to Allergies by Theron G. Randolph, M.D., and Ralph W. Moss, Ph.D. (New York, NY: Bantam Books, 4th edition, 1987).

Coping With Your Allergies by Natalie Golos and Frances Golos

Golbitz (New York: Simon and Schuster, Inc., revised edition, 1986).

Dr. Braly's Food Allergy and Nutrition Revolution by James Braly, M.D. (New Canaan, CT: Keats Publishing, Inc., 1992).

Food Allergies Made Simple by Phylis Austin, Agatha Thrash, M.D., and Calvin Thrash, M.D. (Sunfield, MI: Family Health Publications, 1985).

No More Allergies by Gary Null (New York: Villard Books, 1992).

Tracking Down Hidden Food Allergies by William G. Crook, M.D. (Jackson, TN: Professional Books, 8th printing, 1991).

NOTE
1. Theron G. Randolph and Ralph W. Moss, *An Alternative Approach to Allergies* (New York, NY: Bantam Books, 4th edition, 1987), page 20.

NUTRITION AND ARTHRITIS

INTRODUCTION TO ARTHRITIS

The word *arthritis* comes from the Greek terms *arthron* (joint) and *itis* (inflammation). Arthritis, then, is an inflammation of the joints. There are twenty different kinds of arthritis. Some affect the bones; some, just the joints. Some of the labels that one hears most often include gout, osteoarthritis, rheumatoid arthritis, rheumatism, and osteoporosis.

Bottom line, arthritis is a symptom, not a disease. It's a symptom that all is not well in the human system. As Bernard Jensen, Ph.D. and clinical nutritionist, points out, "All of these conditions come from the same chemical shortages in the body."[1]

The Jensen method of approaching the treatment of rheumatism, arthritis, and osteoporosis is to use food and lifestyle changes as medicine. "You must understand this idea before you can be well," writes Dr. Jensen. "You can use drugs to take away symptoms temporarily, but only foods can change your body to get rid of the cause of the problem. New tissue can be developed best with proper nutritional means."

Contained here are the stories of four people who followed the lead of Jensen and others as they learned how to win back their health through nutritional means.

NANCY BENTLEY

All around her were the sights and sounds of chaos—broken glass, mangled metal, people shouting, sirens screaming, black smoke billowing thick into the clear Iowa sky. Nancy Bentley stood at the side of the road trembling. The child she clutched in her arms was frightened and crying.

Moments earlier, she'd been a passenger in her mother's car. As they approached a pocket of road construction, the flagman had signaled their car to a halt, along with several others. Husband Allen was following in their car.

Reaching into the back, Nancy unfastened her son from the child seat. As long as they had to wait, she might as well feed him. He'd been getting fussy.

Suddenly, and without warning, there was an explosion, like someone had set off an atom bomb nearby. What followed was a horrible, awful screeching sound, as if a million fingernails had been scratched across a single chalkboard. It was the kind of thing that would set your hair on end for life. In a sort of eerie slow motion, Nancy felt her body rolling and pitching and tumbling.

Witnessing the scene that day, you would have wondered how anyone could have escaped unharmed. A huge semi-truck had plowed into the back end of the last car in line. Whether he'd lost his brakes or fallen asleep at the wheel was never really clear. In a deadly game of dominoes, one car piled into the next. Allen's vehicle had smashed his mother-in-law's; and hers, into the one ahead. One car after another was crushed or tumbled into the ditch below. As the line of stunned and wounded motorists waited helplessly for the authorities to arrive, the eighteen-wheeler burst into flames. Amazingly, the Bentleys and Nancy's mother were unharmed.

A month later, as life seemed to be returning to a semblance of normalcy, Nancy noticed a growing pain and swelling in her joints, particularly her hands and knees. In fact, her whole body felt sore. And she was always tired. A rheumatologist was consulted. His diagnosis—rheumatoid arthritis (RA), the bad one. Not only does it involve pain in the joints and connective tissues, like the more mild osteoarthritis, but the whole body is affected.

RA brings stiffness, swelling, fatigue, anemia, weight loss, fever, and often skeletal crippling.

"The doctor prescribed medication," recalls Nancy. "I took it for several weeks but saw no relief in symptoms. He then suggested surgery as an option—taking out the lining of my knees, then letting them grow back. Oh, my, I just knew there had to be a better way."

With a college degree in nutrition to her credit, Nancy was quick to consider that perhaps diet played a key role in her problems with arthritis. She went to see a clinical ecologist who tested her for food and chemical allergies. Results showed that she was allergic not only to corn, yeast, chocolate, dairy products, and sugar, but had probably received an overload of toxic chemicals from breathing in the fumes from the burning truck at the scene of the accident. She would have to adjust her eating habits, as well as avoid anything in her home that gave off toxic fumes. Her gas oven was the first thing to go.

Eager to do all she could to win back her health—all, that is, except drugs and surgery—Nancy followed this advice. But she didn't stop there. She began to add to her battle plan anything and everything that she heard had helped others.

"If someone said that something had worked for them or others, I'd think, *Why not try it?* I read everything I could get my hands on. I read Paavo Airola's book *There Is a Cure For Arthritis*, and I made further changes to my already restrictive diet. No meat, no dairy. Lots of raw, organic fruits and vegetables. I read Bernard Jensen's book *Tissue Cleansing Through Bowel Management* and went on a juice fast. I also began doing enemas to help flush my liver and colon of toxins and parasites. During one enema I actually flushed thirty worms out of my system. This sounds gross, but I called my husband into the bathroom to come see them. You could actually tell which end was the head. Obviously my immune system had not been strong enough to destroy them inside my intestines. My doctor put me on a "de-wormer," and I did garlic enemas, which many consider effective against parasites.

"The interesting thing I discovered about my colon while doing the enemas was that I had been chronically constipated for my entire life. I had what is referred to as an 'anterior anus.' Normally, feces from the large intestine drop into the rectum before being excreted. Mine didn't have to. My bowels were packed all the way down to my rectum all the time. No wonder when I'd gone in for a physical, the doctor would always say, 'You really should move your bowels before you have this exam.' I had no idea.

Doing the enemas helped to restore lost muscle tone in that part of my colon. I remember the first time I felt the feces drop into my rectum. I thought, *Wow, this is something I haven't felt before.*

"I did other things to promote health, too. Besides the fasting, the strict diet, and the enemas, I began to swim regularly. Exercise is essential for reducing pain and retarding joint deterioration. I also got some professional counseling. I'd heard that emotional stress could be a contributing factor to the onset of symptoms. When you talk about health issues, you can't divide one part of the body from the rest. I was dealing with a lot of guilt for having taken my son out of the car seat just before the accident. Dealing with my emotional health was important to winning back my physical health."

Did all these things help Nancy win back her health?

"Oh, yes," she recalls. "It took about a year, but it did turn around."

There seem to have been so many potential contributors to the onset of her condition. Did bowel problems and diet really play a significant role?

"Absolutely," she says, with the assurance of someone who knows what she's talking about. "My major in school was nutrition. I'm not much of a cook, but I love to study and do research about how food affects our bodies. If a person is constipated, his bowel absorbs back into the bloodstream what the body was trying to get rid of. If part of this reabsorption includes proteins that have not been broken down, the body will say, 'What's this?' and set up an immune response. A lot of arthritic symptoms can be traced to this sort of problem."

And what about diet?

"When I first got sick, I went to the clinic here to do some research. It just happens that I live in Rochester, Minnesota, home of the Mayo Clinic. The scientific literature definitely points toward there being a 'gut' component to arthritis. The American College of Rheumatology used to say that diet had no impact upon arthritis. They're beginning to change their tune. Now they're acknowledging that food can affect the body positively, enhancing the functioning of the immune system, or negatively, by evoking an allergic response. They're saying that perhaps 20 percent of those dealing with arthritis are experiencing an allergic reaction to foods. Personally, I think the percentage is much higher. But even so, they've opened the door. For so long they told people that there's absolutely no relationship between foods and arthritis. They labeled such thinking "quackery." However, the research was overwhelming when they did studies on people. Another organization, the American Arthritis Foundation, is in the process of rewriting their position on diet as well."

Nancy has fought back against the debilitating impact of rheumatoid arthritis not once, but twice. Five years after her first bout, it returned with a vengeance.

"The second time around it was in most every joint in my body," she recalls with a wince. "I hurt so much that I spent most of my days lying on the couch. I couldn't lift the basket to do laundry. It hurt my feet to drive. I couldn't have opened the car door, anyhow. I couldn't cook or do any of my tasks around the house. Allen would go to work, then come home and do my work as well. We had three kids at the time. The stress on our family was significant."

What brought it on the second time?

"Probably a combination of things. It's interesting that both flareups came in the fall, a time of year when the gas heat gets turned on in our house. I'd also been told not to get my hair permed—that the chemicals (formaldehyde) involved would be too much for my body to take. But I thought I had gotten to the point where my immune system could handle it, so I got my hair done. The neighbors next door had also been spraying chemicals on their trees. Added to all that, Allen and I were experiencing some rough waters in our relationship. The chemicals and the stress, plus the fact that I wasn't following my diet the way I should've been. . . . I have no doubt that it all mounted up to bring back the symptoms."

Nancy had been a real fighter the first time around. What about the second?

"When it came back I experienced an overwhelming sense of grief. I thought I had beaten it for good and that it would never return. I had to admit to myself that maybe this wasn't just a temporary thing. The first time you whip the dragon, you feel victorious. I guess I was sort of cocky. Now I knew that this was something I would always have to deal with on a regular basis. I found myself disappearing. It sent me to my knees. I remember crying out to God, 'What do you want me to do? You name it.' I got into this whole 'bargaining' thing. 'If you'll take this away, I'll do this and that for you.'

"I was able to turn it around the second time by getting back on the strict diet, and I also added herbs to my battle plan. I read a book called *God's Pharmacy*, which recommended Swedish bitters as a helpful herb for arthritis. I also found a chiropractor who got me on some very good vitamins and supplements, plus did muscle response testing on me to check for an even wider range of food allergies. The first time around the clinical ecologist was able to try only a few foods at a time because of his sublingual (under the tongue) method of testing.

"I also started getting total body massage. It was wonderful! The therapist worked the swelling in my joints and got the fluids moving, sort of 'jump starting' the electrical system in my body. And having someone spend all that time working on me really gave me an emotional boost."

Obviously, Nancy took a different path than that recommended by her original rheumatologist. Did he or anyone else ever think she was nuts?

"Are you kidding? I live in Rochester, Minnesota. We're talking about conservative medicine city here. All my friends work at the Mayo Clinic. They didn't just think I was an oddball, they were angry with me. My best friend said, 'You're just so stupid!' She had to distance herself from me. People don't like to see those they love in pain, and they figure the doctor is the only way to make the pain go away. If they're uncomfortable with what you're doing to treat your problem, they won't always rally behind you. That's hard to take." Even Nancy's family members have been skeptical about her approach. "They still think that I'm a bit wacky, but since I've gotten better, they're feeling more comfortable with my views on health and diet."

Today Nancy Bentley is doing well and going strong. Every chance she gets, she tries to influence people along nutritional lines. "It just bothers me," she admits, "when I see people ignoring the facts. There is indeed a solid link between diet and arthritis."

HELEN BALYEAT

Could it actually be that Helen Balyeat has exchanged her wheelchair for a pair of skis?! Ten years ago the potential of such a thing happening would have been improbable, impossible, absurd. Seventy-year-old ladies crippled with arthritis in their shoulders, hands, and feet should think twice about going up stairs, much less down mountains. And yet. . . .

"I'd had arthritis for years," Helen recalls. "But when I hit sixty it really came hard, mostly in my feet. My bones started to deteriorate rapidly. For about a year I was immobilized. It was a crushing blow to be told by the doctors that there was nothing more they could do."

Arthritis had been no stranger to the clan from which Helen had come. Her mother had been wheelchair-bound for years with the same crippling disease. That debilitating pain and frustration was not something Helen wished to relive.

"The doctors were telling us, 'Get the wheelchair; just get the chair, and get on with the rest of your life.' But I told them, 'Nope, I'm not ready to give in yet.'" And indeed, she wasn't. With the spirit of a captain unwilling to see her ship go down without a fight, she set about to see what could be done to keep her legs beneath her.

"I started going from doctor to doctor, trying to find an alternative to giving up walking. Along the way I found a shop that built me a special pair of shoes. The folks there were very compassionate, willing to take the time to listen to my problem. The wonderful shoes they designed gave me just the kind of support I needed to keep using my feet."

Helen also found out about improving her diet. "I'd been interested in nutrition for some time but hadn't done anything about it," she confesses. "You tend to get serious when the pain starts to get serious." After reading some books by Dr. Paavo Airola about diet and arthritis, she began to see in her own health the correlation between animal products on her menu and pain in her joints and bones. "As a result, I got off all meat and dairy and started juicing fruits and vegetables." She also takes dietary supplements to help meet the operational demands of her system. "At my nutritionist's suggestion, I recently added more minerals and vitamin B_6."

Daily exercise also became part of Helen's battle plan to win back her health. "My husband and I walk a couple of miles every day. To our delight, we've located a doctor in our area who feels the same way we do about diet and exercise. Not only has he been helping me with my problems, but he's working with my husband to rebuild nutritionally after radiation and chemo for lung cancer."

Recently, Helen went in for a bone scan to see how things were going. No further deterioration was found. "It's better in my hands. It's better in my shoulders. It's better everywhere. I'm just convinced that when it comes to fighting degenerative disease, nutrition and exercise are the way to go!" And she's been telling her friends. "I have three friends with cancer. I've told all of them about what I've learned about nutrition. Two elected not to try it, the third did. The first two are going downhill; the third is doing great."

Talking about going downhill, in the state of Washington people over seventy ski free. Guess who's toying with the idea of hitting the slopes this winter.

"That's right," says Helen, "the shoe store steered me to a foot doctor who was also a ski instructor. He said that with a special pair of boots, I could probably ski again. When winter rolls around, I may just try it."

Whether or not she ever actually dons a pair of skis again, Helen is a winner. Instead of playing helpless victim to a criminal disease that threatens to rob her of her mobility, she has taken charge of her battle and fought back. Not everyone with arthritis will be as successful as Helen, but then not all with arthritis are willing to change their diets and exercise either.

MRS. N

Andrew Weil, M.D., teaches at the University of Arizona College of Medicine, has a private medical practice, and is the author of *Natural Health, Natural Medicine* (Houghton Mifflin, 1990). He shares the following story about one of his arthritic patients.

When Mrs. N came in the door one October morning, I liked her at once. She was seventy, soft-spoken, and obviously deformed by rheumatoid arthritis, yet she radiated warmth and good energy. She told me she'd had rheumatoid arthritis (RA) for more than forty years. RA is an autoimmune disorder in which the immune system attacks the joints; with osteoarthritis, it is wear and tear that damages the joints. RA affects younger people and women more often than men; osteoarthritis affects older people and both sexes equally.

Mrs. N told me that she had a high tolerance for pain and had managed fairly well. I could see that the arthritis was severe: Her hands were stiff and clawed, her shoulders bent, and she moved her head with difficulty. Recently the pain had increased, she said, and her neck had become even less mobile. "We're about to go into winter, and that's usually my worst time. Is there anything your kind of medicine can offer me?"

I was amazed to learn that Mrs. N was not taking any medication other than aspirin, and furthermore, that she had never taken anything other than aspirin during the entire course of her illness. "How can that be?" I asked her. It is unheard of for a patient with RA to go through life on aspirin alone. She answered that many doctors along the way had urged her to take stronger drugs— prednisone, gold, methotrexate, and so on—but her intuitive sense of the dangers of these treatments had led her to refuse them. She repeated that she had a high tolerance for pain and said that until recently, aspirin had given her sufficient relief.

In reviewing her lifestyle, I saw a number of possible changes to suggest. Mrs. N's diet was better than average, but she was eating too much protein, including some red meat, chicken, and dairy products. She used margarine and an all-purpose vegetable oil. Her main exercise was walking. The one area in which she was doing fine was her relationships. She told me that she had a wonderful marriage and a rich family life. As she talked about her husband and their relationship, her happiness became even more visible. Clearly, her marriage was a major source of emotional support and satisfaction that probably accounted in some measure for her ability to tolerate a painful and disabling chronic illness.

Not only had Mrs. N paid little attention to the suggestions made by conventional doctors for the management of rheumatoid arthritis, she had never investigated any alternative treatments. I told her I had many recommendations and thought she might greatly benefit from them if she were willing to experiment. I began with an explanation of the value of a very low-protein diet for RA and other autoimmune conditions. High-protein diets irritate the immune system. I suggested that she eat more starches, fruits, and vegetables and that she try to eliminate milk and milk products from her diet.

I also recommended that she eliminate margarine, all partially hydrogenated fats, and all polyunsaturated vegetable oils, since these products promote inflammation. I told her instead to use quality olive and canola oils, as well as to supplement her diet with one tablespoon of flax oil a day, as a source of omega-3 fatty acids, which reduce inflammation. I asked if she liked sardines. (I have found that many women do not.) She did. I suggested that she eat sardines packed in sardine oil twice a week; these are another source of omega-3's (so are salmon, herring, mackerel, and kippers).

I prescribed a basic antioxidant formula (beta carotene, vitamin C, vitamin E, and selenium) along with vitamin B$_6$ (100 milligrams twice a day) and an herb called "feverfew" (Tanacetum parthenium), which is beneficial in treating RA. (American feverfew products are not always effective. I recommended a certain brand of freeze-dried feverfew leaf.)

Mrs. N did not know about the value of movement in water— water will not traumatize joints and allows them to move freely without the stress of gravity. She had access to a heated pool, and I suggested that she visit it at least three times a week. If she wanted to swim, I told her to use a face mask and snorkel so that she would not have to move her head from side to side in order to breathe.

Finally, I sent her to a qualified hypnotherapist, a clinical psychologist I work with, who shares my belief in the importance of the mind/body connection and who is experienced with the management of autoimmunity. It is a common experience that the ups and downs of autoimmune diseases correlate with emotional ups and downs.

I told Mrs. N that there were other practitioners I could send her to, including an acupuncturist, but that I did not want to overload her with suggestions. This was enough work to keep her busy for quite a while. I told her to be patient, because natural treatments take time to produce noticeable changes, and I asked her to call me in two months with a report on her condition.

She called me six weeks later. "I want you to know you're talking to a very happy woman," she began. "I can't believe how much improvement I've had. The pain is less, I have greater mobility, and this is usually the time of year when I suffer most." I told her I thought the improvement would continue.

I had never seen a patient with rheumatoid arthritis respond so quickly to these interventions. Mrs. N was elderly, and she'd had the disease for a long time. Why did she have such good results?

I can see two reasons. The first is that she had never used the strong suppressive treatments of conventional medicine. As I have often written, these drugs may make symptoms disappear and may be necessary for the short-term management of severe flare-ups, but using them for months and years strengthens the disease process and lessens the chance that it will respond to natural interventions. In fact, this is one argument, aside from the risk of toxicity, for being wary of suppressive therapy.

The second reason for Mrs. N's success has to do with her personality and emotional health. She was genuinely happy in a good marriage; her disease was an annoyance for her, though not the focus of her life. It is a different experience to try to work with patients who are deeply unhappy and unsupported emotionally, even if their illnesses are less severe and ordinarily would be responsive to natural medicine.

I continue to be surprised at the closed-mindedness of rheumatologists toward therapies other than suppressive drugs. It is currently the official position of the Rheumatoid Arthritis Foundation that diet has no effect on the disease, despite research to the contrary and despite increasing evidence of the role of dietary fats in promoting or retarding inflammatory processes. Of course, most M.D.'s know little about vitamin therapy and continue to teach that vitamins have no place in medicine except in minimal dosages to prevent deficiency states. The failure of rheumatologists to recommend mind/body interventions—things like hypnotherapy and guided imagery therapy—to arthritis sufferers is disappointing but not surprising, since a general lack of interest in mind/body interactions is characteristic of orthodox medicine as a whole.

I wish I could promise all patients with rheumatoid arthritis that they would have the kind of dramatic and rapid improvement that Mrs. N experienced, but I can't. RA is variable in its effects, and when very active, may require conventional intervention, including immunosuppressive drugs and corrective surgery. I do think that natural medicine can be of help to all persons with this disease, even in combination with the standard treatments. It may enable them to get by with lower doses of prednisone, for example, or to get off the suppressive drugs more quickly. And for many patients, especially for those with early disease, mild disease, and disease that comes and goes, the treatments I recommended to Mrs. N may be all that is needed to manage the condition.

Dr. James Braly, M.D.

Los Angeles–based physician, researcher, educator, and author of Dr. Braly's Food Allergy and Nutrition Revolution—*The following story is taken from a talk delivered to representatives of Bio Metics, International.*

I started practicing clinical nutrition on a full-time basis and made the decision early on that I would practice medicine without the use of prescription drugs. I did that for a very good reason. I began to see that often changing a person's diet and putting them on supplementation could reverse diseases. Not just prevent disease, but actually reverse it.

I was particularly enamored by the ability of dietary change to reverse some diseases that I was taught in med school were to be treated almost exclusively by drugs. One example would be rheumatoid arthritis (RA).

In the early 1980s I had the good fortune of having the actor James Coburn come into my practice. I can recall that he was so immobilized that his friend Lee Majors, with him at the time, had to help him into the chair in my office. When our appointment was over, Lee had to help James back up out of the chair.

The story that Mr. Coburn told me was that his father had died from the complications of rheumatoid arthritis. It was obvious that he was experiencing symptoms and signs of the same disease. He'd gone to a rheumatologist for help, but basically wasn't getting better on the drugs he'd been prescribed.

To make a long story short, James went on a fast for fifteen days—a water and fresh juice fast. The symptoms of his rheumatoid arthritis disappeared! He then went back to the rheumatologist to discuss what had happened, and perhaps have him design an ongoing program that would keep the disease from reappearing. The doctor's response was a cold, "Well, you can't fast forever." He summarily dismissed any cause-and-effect relationship between diet and arthritic disease.

So that's when James came to my clinic. Through dietary manipulation and supplementation we once again got him into a symptom free state. It took us thirty days. He has remained that way over the last decade.

QUOTES

"All experience and observations—empirical, statistical, and clinical—point out that the causes for degenerative pathological changes leading to arthritis are found in the general deterioration and breakdown of man's resistance. This degeneration is due to his unhealthy, disease-producing, 'civilized' way of life

characterized by: lack of exercise, devitalized diet, poisonous environment, smoking, poisonous drugs, emotional and physical stress, etc. Of these, faulty nutrition is, perhaps, the most significant health-destroying factor."

—Karl-Otto Aly, M.D.
AS QUOTED IN *THERE IS A CURE FOR ARTHRITIS*
BY PAAVO O. AIROLA, N.D.

"Faulty nutrition is singularly the most important causative factor in the development of arthritis. An unbalanced diet of devitalized, over-processed, overcooked, and overrefined denatured foods combined with toxic and foodless items such as tobacco, alcohol, coffee, sugar, salt, irritating spices, chocolate, soft drinks, sweets, pastries, pies, etc., together with other negative environmental factors, brings about a general deterioration of health, biochemical imbalance, and systemic disturbances. These deleterious factors eventually lead to a total metabolic disorder and consequent pathological changes in the joints and tissues of the body."

—Paavo O. Airola, N.D.
THERE IS A CURE FOR ARTHRITIS

"Diet change is the single most beneficial thing you can do to control the causes and symptoms of arthritis."
—Linda Rector Page, N.D., Ph.D.
HEALTHY HEALING

FURTHER READING
Arthritis: Don't Learn to Live With It by Carlton Fredericks, Ph.D. (New York, NY: Perigee Books, 1981).

Arthritis, Rheumatism, and Osteoporosis by Bernard Jensen, Ph.D. (Escondido, CA: Bernard Jensen Enterprises, 1986).

Freedom From Arthritis Thru Nutrition by Philip J. Walsh, D.D.S., N.D., and Bianca Leonardo, N.D. (Joshua Tree, CA: Tree of Life Publications, 1992).

There Is a Cure for Arthritis by Paavo O. Airola, N.D. (West Nyack, NY: Parking Publishing Company, Inc., 1968).

NOTE
1. Bernard Jensen, Ph.D., Clinical Nutritionist, *Arthritis, Rheumatism, and Osteoporosis* (Escondido, CA: Bernard Jensen Enterprises, 1986), pages 1-2.

5

NUTRITION AND CANCER

INTRODUCTION TO CANCER

From the cancer family tree hang the names of as many as 250 types of the disease—colon cancer, breast cancer, lung cancer, and on and on. As you read the stories that follow, you may not find someone who has battled back from the same sort of cancer which you have. From the alternative medicine point of view, that's okay. Cancer, they contend, is a systemic disease—an opportunistic condition that develops in the part of your body that is weakest. It may be weak because of a genetic predisposition or diet or environmental exposures, but because it is that way, that's where cancer finds a foothold in your system.

Keeping that in mind, these stories are presented as representative of fighting cancer, any kind of cancer, from the nutritional point of view.

DAVID BOLSTER

David Bolster sat in a reclining chair watching fluid drip from an IV bag, down a tube, and into his veins. As he leaned back and shut his eyes, his mind relived the events that had brought him to this place.

He and wife, Lawnie, were professional entertainers, singers.

They'd been playing the hotel and casino circuit throughout Nevada for years. He'd been at it for twenty-eight. She, for fifteen.

One day while showering, he'd noticed a lump in the groin area of his left leg. An oversized pimple, he thought. It didn't hurt, but he told his wife. She reminded him about a physical he was scheduled for soon. The lump would be a good thing to ask about.

During the ensuing days, the mysterious lump neither grew nor diminished in size. David didn't pay it much attention. In fact, his concern was so little, that he failed to bring it up during his physical. Returning to the doctor's office later in the week for blood test results, he mentioned it in passing. To his surprise the doctor started probing other areas of his body as well.

"If you were me," the doctor confided, "I wouldn't do anything about it. But you're not me. I want you to see a specialist."

The oncologist David consulted was much more alarmed. "You need to get on chemotherapy immediately!" he ordered in a tone that indicated that he wasn't going to take no for an answer. "You have lymphoma, cancer of the lymph system."

"Can't we think about this for a while?" David pleaded.

"Think about what?" he shot back. "There's nothing to think about! You *must* do this!"

What followed was three months of living hell. Treatments were administered once a week in the oncologist's office, with every fourth time in the hospital. The drugs given that fourth week were so hard on his kidneys that the availability of medical help was required in case there was a need to rescue him from complete shut down.

It was a three-month-long nightmare. His hair fell out, every joint in his body felt like it had been hit with a hammer, his skin felt like it was plastic, and his fingertips ached. The worse part, however, were the marble-sized blisters that developed inside his mouth and on his tongue. Agonizing pain shot through his whole body every time he opened his mouth. Eating or drinking was absolute torture. What little he was able to slide down his throat tasted like metal.

To its credit, the chemotherapy sent his lymphoma into remission. His body slowly began to recover from the onslaught of the poisonous chemicals. Back on the road again, he and Lawnie set out once more to pursue their careers as entertainers. For nearly two years he remained cancer free. Near the end of the second, however, terrible stomach pains and backaches began to rack his body. Tests revealed that a four-by-seven inch cancerous mass had developed in his abdomen.

"We will now do a bone marrow transplant," insisted the same doctor who had earlier pushed chemotherapy on them.

"What are our options?" asked Lawnie.

"Death," replied the doctor, with a certain arrogance in his bluntness that seemed to say, "I am the expert here. Take it, or leave it."

"But can't we just do chemo again?" they pleaded.

The doctor took off his glasses, setting them before him on his desk in a move that was meant to get their complete attention. "Look, the cancer has come back. Chemotherapy has proven ineffective. Your only option if you want to live is to do a bone marrow transplant."

They left his office in tears. They'd done enough research on bone marrow transplants to know that they didn't want any part of that. There had to be another way, but what? David was beginning to lose hope.

The weeks and months that followed were consumed with research. They read everything they could get their hands on concerning alternative cancer therapies. What sort of options were available outside the narrow boundaries of mainstream medicine? Did these therapies have merit? Had others seen success? Where could they go to get this kind of help? How much would it cost? As information kept coming in, prayers kept going out. "God, give us wisdom about what to do."

All the while, David's body continued to swell. The lymphatic mass in his upper abdomen was blocking the flow through his body of essential proteins, enzymes, vitamins, and minerals. The naturopathic physician he was now seeing, with hope of getting nontoxic therapies, suggested that he needed more significant help than she was able to provide. Through her network of information, however, they learned about the American Biologics Clinic in Mexico, a top-notch medical facility dedicated to "alternative" cancer therapies. They also discovered a clinic in Reno, Nevada, called the GAM Diagnostic Nutritional Medical Center, which was offering similar therapies with good results. For cost sake they chose Reno. They also had friends they could stay with.

And here it was that David sat watching fluid drip from an IV bag, down a tube, and into his veins as his mind wandered back over the recent past. It was his fourth day of what would be a three-week series of treatments involving intravenous drips of a mixture of nutrients, including minerals, vitamin C, amino acids, Germanium, and Laetrile. Other people he had met and befriended here were seeing good results.

Suddenly the calm was shattered by heavy footsteps, loud voices, and banging doors. A woman was screaming. Men with P-O-L-I-C-E emblazoned on the back of their jackets were running around inside the clinic. One was barking orders.

"Take the books. Take the computer. Take everything. Leave nothing behind!"

Another voice yelled, "Don't move, and everything will be all right."

A group of paramedics made their way through the commotion in the outer office to the room were David sat with two fellow patients, getting their IV treatments. The three of them just looked at each other in stunned silence. What in the world was happening?!

The paramedics pointed at them and said, "Look, you're free to go, but this place is closed, shut down for good." Without concern for gentleness, the needles were literally jerked from their arms.

For David and Lawnie, it felt like they'd just been raped and plundered. And this by those supposedly dedicated to their protection. In the United States—land of the free, and home of the brave. It was the kind of stuff from which gangster movies and films about Russian politics are fashioned.

The GAM Diagnostic Nutritional Medical Center had been a well-established institution in the community for ten years. Their program of treatment, including their use of Laetrile and other non-toxic therapies, had been listed in John Fink's highly respected

book *Third Opinion*, an international directory to alternative therapy centers for cancer. The woman who ran it, Vera Allison, was
not some shifty shyster out to separate vulnerable people from their
life savings for treatment with placebos and snake oils. She was
a woman of high integrity, a devoted Christian, educated and
licensed as a naturopathic physician from the Pacific College of
Naturopathic Medicine in southern California, and she had been
treating patients for over thirty years.

So, why was this clinic shut down? David and Lawnie never
did find out for sure. An account they read somewhere indicated
that it was politically motivated. The war against health-care "alternatives" rages on. From what they'd been reading about the "strong
arm" antics of some in position to influence health-care policy,
they knew they'd just been knocked out by medical bigotry. If
you're getting better but not by our rules, then we don't want
you getting better.

Another patient had been making steady improvement. Things
looked as if they were going to turn around for him. However,
shortly after the clinic was closed, he died. His link to the kind
of help he needed and wanted had been severed.

Tired and badly shaken, the Bolster's drove to nearby Sacramento, California, to stay a few days with David's brother to
sort things out. David's condition worsened. The fluid collecting
in his abdomen pushed against his lungs and impaired his breathing. A trip to the local hospital, and a procedure to drain the stomach, netted seven liters of fluid! The doctor on duty was full of
doom and gloom. As if he thought himself God, he let them know
right off the bat that David had only about two weeks to live. Even
so, he wished to keep him in the hospital to run more tests and
pump him full of drugs. What sense did that make?

At that point in their journey toward healing, Mexico came
back into the picture. With a bit of financial maneuvering and a lot
of prayer, they managed to scrape together enough money to get
to American Biologics. Was it worth it?

"Oh mercy, yes!" says David emphatically. "It gave me a whole
new lease on life. I lost forty pounds of fluid in three weeks. Their
approach is to take extensive blood tests and analyze your whole

metabolic system to see what your body is missing—what vitamins, minerals, and enzymes it needs to rebuild itself to function the way it was designed to function. I'm convinced that our bodies are designed by God to be self-healing over things like cancer if we provide them with the right nutritional tools.

"Then they design a program of diet, supplements, and other nontoxic therapies tailormade to the individual to help restore his body. In other words, they build up the body to fight off the disease, as opposed to treating the disease itself. The latter is the approach here in the U.S. We cut, burn, and poison in hopes of getting the cancer out. To me, that doesn't make any sense at all.

"American Biologics doesn't use any drugs, unless one would consider Laetrile a drug. It isn't, of course. It's actually a plant-derived nutrient called *amygdalin* or vitamin B_{17}. Why it's banned in the U.S., I really don't quite understand. Perhaps that's why the Reno clinic had been shut down.

"Was our time in Mexico worth it? You be the judge. I went into the hospital in Sacramento sick, it cost me $18,000 for a one-week stay, the doctor gave me no hope, and I left there very sick and discouraged. I went immediately from there to the American Biologic Clinic in Mexico, barely hanging on to life and in a wheelchair. It cost me $10,000 for three weeks of treatment, the whole environment is upbeat and hopeful, and by the time I left I was riding an exercise bike and taking stairs on my own.

David is not out of the woods yet in his battle with lymphoma. There remains much work to be done toward reversing his condition. However, he has found a way to blend together conventional and nutritional therapies into a sort of synergistic teamwork that has his cancer on the run. A local immunologist, sensitive to David's negative feelings about aggressive chemotherapy, has been administering very small doses. To this, David adds juicing (raw fruits and vegetables), a vegetarian diet (no meat or dairy), megadoses of vitamin C, and coffee enemas to keep his liver detoxified.

What would he say to others who are considering their options as they formulate their own cancer battle plan?

"If I knew then what I know now, I never would've done those first three months of intense chemotherapy. I truly believe that cancer is a matter of nutritional deficiency. If I'd been aware of nutritional help when I was originally diagnosed, I certainly would've gone that route right off the bat."

HARRIET DAVIDSON

What was wrong with Harriet Davidson? No one knew.

It all began fourteen years ago when she experienced pain in her right side accompanied by a terrible case of gas—or at least it felt like gas. "When the symptoms first appeared," she remembers, "I noted that many of the customers in my beauty shop were complaining of similar aches and pains. I just chalked it up to some kind of bug that was going around."

But as her patrons got better, Harriet got worse. She became concerned. What was this constant pain in her gut? It just so happened that the local health department was giving out colon kits. Using them, a person could check to see if there was blood in their stool, a potential sign of colon cancer. Harriet tried it twice. Each time she got the same results. Positive.

"The Health Department called," she recalls. "They emphasized that this didn't necessarily mean that I had cancer, but it did indicate that I had internal bleeding that warranted further examination."

At the earliest possible moment, Harriet beat a path to the local health clinic. "Spastic colon" said the doctors who examined her. They gave her a prescription for drugs to relax her muscles and sent her on her way.

It didn't help. A few months later she returned, blood still in her stool. This time they decided that what she really had was a hiatal hernia. "I asked about the bleeding, and they said that both a spastic colon and a hiatal hernia could cause blood in the stool." The doctors, however, performed no tests to verify their diagnosis. They never tried to determine where the bleeding might be coming from. "I now know," says Harriet, a more informed health-care consumer, "that they were just plain careless."

Meanwhile, Harriet's health and stamina were slipping steadily out of control as the pain in her side grew more and more intense. "I would get up in the middle of almost every night to give myself an enema. I thought maybe that would help the gas." Little did she know that the gas pains she was feeling were a byproduct of cancer doing its thing there in her large intestine, eating away at the lining.

"One morning I asked my husband to feel the lump on my side. He thought it was just a roll of fat. But I'd never been overweight. In fact, I'd recently lost nineteen pounds. Besides, a roll of fat shouldn't be hurting like that, should it? I was beginning to suspect that this was *more* than just a spastic colon or a hiatal hernia."

Just how much more was about to be discovered. One night, soon thereafter, Harriet found herself sprawled out like a limp noodle on the cold tile floor of their bathroom. She'd fallen and couldn't get up. Her husband had to come to her rescue, lifting her back to bed. The next morning Harriet found herself almost totally incapacitated. None of the body parts she needed to get herself up and going were working right. An emergency trip to the hospital ensued.

Finally, after months of pain and frustration, the puzzle of what ailed Harriet Davidson was solved. Cancer. A great deal more than the doctors thought. A *great* deal more! And before it was all over, a grapefruit-sized tumor had been removed from her colon.

"When my surgeon came into my hospital room following the surgery, he said, 'Now we want you to do eighteen months of chemotherapy.' The tumor had broken through the intestinal wall and spread to other organs." Sixteen inches of her colon needed to be knifed out, along with a fallopian tube, several lymph nodes, and some of the surrounding fatty tissue. There was no talk of having "gotten it all." Just as well, for that phrase is used far too often by surgeons to give unwarranted comfort to people who actually need to keep their guard up rather than let it down. Whenever there is a tumor big enough to be detected by touch, it's a pretty safe bet that cancer cells have been circulating in the body for some time. Harriet was no exception. It was probably just a matter of time before more tumors would form, unless something was done to prevent this. Chemo was SOP—standard operating procedure.

"I just told him no way! My surgeon was a wonderfully kind doctor, and understanding. But I'd read too much about chemotherapy to want that stuff in my body. It may kill a few cancer cells, but it destroys good cells as well. In the process, the immune system is destroyed, leaving the body nothing left to fight with."

Instead of chemo, Harriet did something that many might consider nuts. "I called a friend at a local health-food store. She gave me some ideas on how to detoxify my liver and build up my immune system. She also gave me the name of a nutritionist who could help."

That was nearly a decade and a half ago. Today Harriet's back at the shop doing hair and telling war stories. "The doctors keep doing tests on me and just shake their heads," she says with the air of someone who has found the needle in the haystack that others overlooked. It's obvious the doctors didn't expect her to live as long as she has, especially without chemotherapy. "They say I'm just lucky."

The prize in the pile of cancer therapies that Harriet Davidson found—which seems to have played such a significant role along with surgery in her own cancer battle plan—has been nutrition. To those who ask, she hands a two-page outline entitled "My Metabolic Diet." Here's a summary of what she did to rebuild her body's own defense systems to ward off recurrent cancer:

Things to Avoid
▲ refined foods (white sugar, white flour, white rice)
▲ fried foods
▲ microwaved foods (too much radiation, causes free radicals to be formed in food that can damage tissue)
▲ food cooked on Teflon-coated cookware (chemicals can be absorbed into body)
▲ red meat (eat fish or chicken once a week if you wish, but you can get enough protein from nuts, beans, and vegetables)
▲ food that has been treated with chemicals (pesticides, herbicides, etc.)

Things to Consume

▲ fiber cleanse (helps to keep colon clean—in particular, she uses wheat grass tablets)

▲ fresh, raw fruits, vegetables, and grains (provide the body with all the nutrients needed)

▲ Pau 'D Arco tea, red clover tea, comfrey tea (taken throughout the day, to help clean the blood)

▲ lots of carrot juice (juice carrots with a green vegetable like Romaine lettuce or green pepper)

▲ purified or distilled water

▲ vitamins A, B, C, E and digestive enzymes (at every meal)

"I recently lost a twenty-six-year-old grandson to cancer," Harriet sadly admits. "He wouldn't listen to me. He was in the service and just followed along with everything the Army doctors wanted to do to him. They told him that I'd been lucky—that what I did wouldn't do a bit of good for him. They killed him with double shots of chemotherapy and then a bone marrow transplant. He left behind two little daughters, three and four years old."

In Harriet's mind, more than luck has brought her back from the edge of death. "Without the surgery to get the big stuff, nutrition to detoxify my body and rebuild my immune power, and the help of God, I wouldn't be alive today," she concludes.

We're listening, Harriet. We're listening.

IRENE ROYBAL

"I was at work one day, and all of a sudden I got a real sharp pain in my left side, just beneath my ribs," recalls Irene Roybal. "I got myself home, and by the time my husband, Tano, got there, the pain had me thrashing around in bed."

What was going on? Where did all this pain come from? She'd always, always been a very active person. Lately, however, she'd been slowing down. In fact, when she came home from work she'd be ready to go right to bed for the night.

"It was getting so I was real tired all the time. Just walking through my house would wear me out. That's not me." Even so, neither she nor Tano gave her falling energy level much thought. But now there was this pain. Might the two be connected?

Tests were run in the local hospital—several days' worth. Finally, the doctors found something in her intestine; something that the rest of us hope and pray will never be found in our intestines—or anywhere else, for that matter. It was the "beast." The Big C. Cancer. And it had perforated her bowel.

After the lab had a chance with the biopsy material to probe and weigh (or whatever lab folks do), they came to the conclusion that this particular brand of the disease had not originated in her small intestine. In other words (gulp!) this was not the primary source of her troubles. Somewhere else in her body, somewhere previously overlooked, the evil menace was quietly at work subverting her immune system and sending out raiding parties to reap havoc on other organs.

"So they gave me more CAT scans, and they found it in my right lung." This, they said, was a primary site. The doctors set about their whittling. By the time they were done, two-thirds of her lung was gone.

When a person starts to lose body parts to a surgeon's knife, they sincerely hope (*very* sincerely!) that whatever problem called for such a drastic solution will come to a satisfactory resolve. Just like anyone else, Irene held such a sincere hope. Three months later, however, the beast showed its ugly head once again. This time in her pancreas. There are bad places for cancer to be. The pancreas is among the most troublesome.

"They took one look at that," recalls Irene of the doctors, "and said there was nothing more they could do. Chemo and surgery wouldn't help."

So as conventionally trained doctors are prone to do when the tools they've been trained to work with no longer help, they handed her a death sentence. In other words, if we can't help you, nobody can. "Mrs. Roybal, we're sorry to have to inform you of this, but you have nine months, tops."

What would you do after being handed your head in your hands like that? Hit a doctor? Jump off a bridge? Drink yourself into oblivion? Irene chose the only response that made sense to her, a response that gave her comfort and peace. "I just told God to take me into his hands, and to do whatever his will was for me, and I'd do what I could down here." A simple faith. A profound surrender. A calm peace. And new direction.

"My husband was driving home from the hospital one day and heard Anne Frähm on John Neider's radio show. She was talking about her own battle with cancer and how she'd ultimately turned the tide through nutrition. He bought *A Cancer Battle Plan*, read it, and by the time I was ready to come home from the hospital had purchased a juicer and everything else, and got me right on the same things that she did."

Now we don't offer *A Cancer Battle Plan* as a blueprint for others to follow. It's our story of what worked for Anne. But the principles underlying what we did would seem to hold true for anyone battling degenerative disease. There are two. First, clean out the body. Get rid of toxic buildup that's been gathering in various organs and cells from diet and environmental causes. That buildup is a terrible drain on the various systems of the body, particularly the immune system, leaving it weak against renegade cells known as cancer. Second, rebuild and enhance the functioning of the key systems. And again, the immune system in particular.

These were the principles that Irene took from our experience and applied to her own. "I did a two-week cleansing diet—taking in only freshly juiced organic fruit and vegetables, while doing enemas to flush toxins. I then began eating vegetarian, exactly as the book described. I also bought Marilyn and Harold Diamond's book *Fit for Life*, and added some of their dietary recommendations. And I've been doing a bunch of the same supplements Anne did. Vitamins A, C, E, pancreatic enzymes, selenium, KYO-Green, Melaluca oil, and Essiac Tea, to name a few."

Would you believe it's been nearly two years since Irene was told she was a goner, and yet she's doing great! People have been taking notice. "The folks in the health-food store see how I'm doing and refer other people to me for encouragement. Right away I tell them about *A Cancer Battle Plan*. But you know, there are a lot of people who just don't want to work through a whole process to get better. I can't believe they're not willing to do whatever it takes to get better, but they're not."

We've met people like that too, Irene. We're glad you're not one of them.

BEATA BISHOP

In 1959 a pioneer in diet therapy against cancer died. His name was Max Gerson. In the pre-war years of the 1930s, Gerson became lasting friends with a Nobel Prize winning colleague by the name of Albert Schweitzer, by curing his wife Helena Schweitzer of lung tuberculosis after conventional medicine had failed to be of help. In 1934 Gerson published a book entitled *Diet Therapy for Lung Tuberculosis* in which Mrs. Schweitzer's recovery was one among many documented. Over the years Dr. Schweitzer followed Gerson's work as his diet therapy was applied to a growing list of pathologies, including heart and kidney failure, and finally cancer. Schweitzer's own adult onset diabetes responded to Gerson's dietary treatment.

Although Dr. Gerson was privileged to testify before a congressional subcommittee as to his work with cancer patients, at that time in the history of modern medicine few cared to hear about the results he was having through something so simple as dietary changes. "Wonder" drugs were emerging on the scene. Medical technology was booming. Together these were going to cure the world of sickness and disease. Or so we thought.

At his death, Gerson was eulogized by friend Albert Schweitzer: "I see in him one of the most eminent geniuses in the history of medicine. Many of his basic ideas have been adopted without having his name connected with them. Yet he has achieved more than seemed possible under adverse conditions. He leaves a legacy which commands attention and which will assure him his due place. Those whom he cured will now attest to the truth of his ideas."[1]

Truth is, during his life he received far less respect for his work than he's getting now as the list of people grows who have successfully used his therapy to win back their health from the clutches of cancer. One of the names on that list is a Londoner named Beata

Bishop, who wrote her own book entitled *My Triumph Over Cancer*. What follows is a portion of a letter we recently received from her, briefly outlining her own cancer battle plan.

"In November of 1979 I was diagnosed with malignant melanoma. I had a small tumor on my right shin. The orthodox treatment was surgery, a wide excision on my right leg, with a skin graft. The operation was apparently a success, but it left me with months of pain, impeded movement, and horribly mutilated.

"In December of 1980 a hard lymph node was found in my right groin. By then I had done my own research into malignant melanoma and realized that the cancer had spread into the lymph system. This was very bad news, indeed. The surgeon suggested another operation to remove the lymph glands in my right groin, and anything else that might be affected. I did not see how a second operation could solve the problem when the first one did not, and so refused further surgery.

"At the same time, I found out through a friend about the Gerson therapy. Having read his book in record time, I was struck by the clarity and logic of his therapy and decided to try it. The essence of it is this: People don't get cancer unless their metabolism is severely damaged, their system becomes highly toxic, and their immune system does not work properly. Therefore, to cure an existing cancer, patients need to be thoroughly detoxified and given optimum hyper-nutrition in order to restore their metabolism and their immune system to full functioning. Once the body has been brought back to optimum condition and functioning, it can get rid of the malignant process that has manifested in the shape of one or more tumors.

"This is where the Gerson therapy radically differs from conventional cancer treatments: (1) It sees the tumor not as the disease, but as the symptom of a deep underlying cause—i.e., a dysfunctional system, as detailed above; and (2) it aims to restore the entire body so that it can heal itself, instead of concentrating on removing or destroying the tumor. Above all, instead of using aggressive, invasive, and/or toxic methods—such as surgery, radiation, and chemotherapy—this therapy works gently and nontoxically *with* the body.

"All this is done by putting the patient on an organic vegetarian diet for a year and a half or two—salt-free and fat-free, with a large intake of freshly made fruit and vegetable juices (thirteen eight-ounce glasses a day, one every hour on the hour). Detoxification is promoted by frequent coffee enemas (up to five a day at first, then gradually diminishing) and the use of castor oil. Medication consists of natural substances, the only purpose of which is to improve digestion and produce a potassium-sodium balance in the body.

"I entered the Gerson clinic near Tijuana, Mexico, in January of 1981, and stayed there for eight weeks before returning to London. I continued on the intensive therapy for another sixteen months, and on a less strict program for another six months. At the very beginning, my mild diabetes disappeared, never to return, and the incipient osteoarthritis in my right hand also vanished. After some six weeks, the surgically mutilated part of my right leg began to grow back some flesh, and eventually replaced nearly 50 percent of the loss. These early results encouraged me to persevere with the lengthy, monotonous, labor-intensive, and frankly boring therapy.

"Having been given six weeks to six months to live by my surgeon in December of 1980 if I refused a further operation, and being in good health thirteen years later, I consider that I made the right choice in those dark and desperate days so long ago.

"Nutrition was the sole determining factor in my recovery. During the second year of the therapy I had weekly reflexology sessions with an outstanding therapist. I do believe that they helped me, too. As a psychotherapist, I realize that my level of stress and state of mind during the one or two years preceding my illness played a part in undermining my immune system . . . and during my recovery I did receive occasional counseling. In no way do I underestimate the role of the psyche in sickness and health, but for myself I feel sure that without the brilliant nutritional approach of the Gerson therapy, I would not be alive today.

"And I'm very alive, indeed! I have a high level of energy and an increased capacity for enjoyment. I am trying to repay my debt by helping others who are on the therapy and by trying to persuade open-minded doctors to take a good look at the importance of nutrition in the cancer-fighting field. Some of them actually seem to listen."

WILLIAM "BILL" D. CARSON

All blood. That's what Bill Carson's urine looked like. Tests were performed, including the one men fear most—a tube inserted through the opening in the penis into the bladder. Cringe! Thank goodness for anesthesia!

"When the doctor came into my hospital room with the results," recalls Bill, "I was not too surprised to learn that I had a malignant tumor in my bladder. Cancer. It was growing directly on the lining, with indications that it had invaded the muscle wall. That meant it was a good bet that the cancer had spread to the lymph glands and could ultimately spread throughout my body."

"It's stage four," the doctor had said, "the angry kind. That means it can spread quickly. In these situations, it's best to remove the bladder."

Imagine life with a bag glued to your front to collect urine. That was the future Bill was facing if he did what the doctors thought best. The operation is called a cystectomy. Because the bladder is removed, a substitute to store urine is needed. In the method most often used, a small segment of the small intestines is converted into a conduit, or pipeline, for urine. The ureters—tubes that carry urine from each kidney to the bladder—are joined to one end of the segment. The other end is brought out through the wall of the abdomen, near the navel, where it forms an opening called a *stoma*. That's where the bag is attached, right over that stoma.

The medical types wanted to rush Bill to the major hospital in the area and get after his bladder. "My scheduled arrival was within ten days, and my bladder was to be removed within thirteen," he recalls.

Imagine the flood of questions and fears you'd have if you were in his shoes. A person needs time to think about their options when faced with amputation of body parts. These things don't grow on trees, you know! Once gone, always gone.

Bill asked if they could remove just a section of the bladder and save the function of the rest. "In order to be safe," replied his doctors, "it would be best to have the whole bladder removed. This would assure coverage if the malignancy had spread throughout the muscle of the bladder. Furthermore, if other organs had been affected, they too could be removed."

Both his urologist and internist insisted that this was the proper thing to do medically, and for his own good. He would also need to have any other organs cut out that had been affected, and he would have to live out the rest of his life glued to a bag. No other alternatives were suggested. Black and white. Cut and dried.

That's when a friend with a simple story suggested that there might be a better way. He had been diagnosed some eight years earlier with 98 percent blockage in three of his arteries and had not been expected to live more than a week or two. In an effort to save his own life, he'd gotten hooked up with a doctor who did chelation therapy—a safe, painless, nonsurgical method of removing obstructive plaque from the circulatory system via an intravenous drip of certain amino acids and nutrients. And here he was, by golly, still alive and kicking to tell about it years later. Maybe this kind of thing would help Bill.

"I found out," recalls Bill, "that this doctor my friend saw operated a clinic at that time in Alabama and made it his practice to treat the whole patient—physically, mentally, and spiritually. He was a devout Christian and defined his practice of medicine as 'wholistic.'"

Intrigued and hopeful, Bill sought him out. With the belief in God as a common bond, a predisposition toward nutrition and natural medicine, and a definite desire not to have his body cut up, he cast his lot with the good doctor to see what might be done.

"My treatments began with the chelation therapy, and in my case included 50,000 milligrams of vitamin C daily for twenty-six days. Also included in the chelation drip were vitamin B_{15}, which increased cellular oxidation, and vitamin B_{17}, otherwise known as Amygdalin or Laetrile, which appears to be fatal to cancer cells."

In addition, Bill received the following therapies:

▲ Hyperbaric oxygen (HBO) therapy, which increases the blood's oxygen content and enhances the effectiveness of chelation
▲ Detoxification and colon therapy to rid the body of poisons and accumulated toxins
▲ Hydrotherapy for preventive physical maintenance
▲ Physical therapy for muscular, circulation, and nerve conditioning
▲ Exercise
▲ Enzyme therapy (pancreatic, digestive, proteolytic), which facilitates chemical reactions that fight and dissolve cancer cells
▲ Vitamins A and E
▲ Plus other possible aids to cancer remission, like special teas, bee pollen, AlphLac, and inositol tablets

Within twenty days, Bill's cancer was gone! No trace of it was left in his body. That was over six years ago. Today X-rays show a clear bladder. Blood and urine tests show no living cancer cells. And just think, he could be wearing a bag and wondering what body parts he'd be missing next!

As a result of all that he'd learned and experienced, Bill left behind his forty-year commercial banking career, wrote a book entitled *Six Months to Life*, and has dedicated the rest of his days to helping people battle back from degenerative disease by means of nontoxic, non-invasive therapies and nutrition. Before long, he found himself in the employment of Dr. Evers, the doctor who had helped him so much, who was in the midst of launching a new clinic in Mexico. He'd been forced out of the U.S. by the "powers that be" in medical politics—namely, the Food and Drug Administration (FDA) and the American Medical Association (AMA). Seems they had a problem with some of the things he was using to help people, in particular vitamin B_{17} (Laetrile) and chelation therapy. Bill was invited to move to El Paso, Texas, with his wife, and help run the U.S. office of what has become known as the International Medical Center (IMC) of Juarez, Mexico.

As an epilogue to Bill's story, he has recently left the IMC and is in the process of starting another clinic in the Juarez area, utilizing the protocols developed and successfully used for years by Dr. Evers and his associates. As for the good doctor himself, he went to meet his Maker in 1990. "He was considered the grandfather of chelation therapy," notes Bill. "We will truly miss this pioneer who gave his life to the healing and treating of humanity."

MAY ENGLES

When May Engles was thirty-eight she found something that scared the heck out of her. A lump. "I was a basket case," she says of those days. "I knew something was wrong with me, but I didn't know what. Then I found this thing in my breast."

In retrospect, May points to stress as the key factor that had over time weakened her immune system and allowed cancer cells to go unchecked in her body. "We'd had some awful things happen. In fact, just one year before finding the lump, our house was burglarized by two ex-con's who had just been released from the local penitentiary. That really hit me hard. I lived with a fear inside of me that was absolutely paralyzing. When I hear experts talking about the mind-body connection—how emotional stress can cause illness—I know exactly what they're talking about. I'm convinced that's what happened to me."

A mastectomy was performed on her left breast. She was relieved to hear that there was no lymph node involvement, that the cancer had not spread. "The next day the surgeon came into my room and told me that the lab had made an unfortunate error. Truth was, nine out of sixteen nodes were involved."

Just what she didn't need to hear. Already devastated by the loss of her breast, May was so low she had to look up to see carpet. Would she be able to beat this stuff? Her doctor was recommending a year of chemotherapy.

About four months into the chemo, she happened to be in a store talking to someone about her situation. A man standing nearby overheard their conversation and interrupted.

"Please get off chemotherapy," he warned. "It's going to end up killing you." And he suggested that she pick up a book entitled

Cancer Winner by Jackie Davison. She did.

"That man and that book convinced me to quit chemo," she admits. "I just threw it all out and decided to look into nutritional therapies. I'd already been feeling as if I was falling apart; that the chemo was destroying me, both physically and emotionally. The conversation with that man sealed it for me. My oncologist thought I really was nuts, of course. When I got my medical records from him to begin looking for a nutritionist, I was stunned. Right there in black and white, he'd written that he thought I was mentally deficient, because I thought nutrition could heal me. I was so upset, I just cried and cried. Here I was trying desperately to build myself back up, and there he was tearing me down."

She cried some more. When she was done, she made a commitment. "In spite of everything, I decided that if I was going to make it, nutrition was going to be the way."

May never did find a nutritionist she was satisfied with. However, here and there she picked up bits and pieces of information of what others had done to win back their own health from cancer. Together she and her husband launched themselves on an adventure in healing. They got a juicer and began flooding her system with fresh, organic juices—carrot, apple, beet, parsley, celery, and cabbage. Fresh salads became a mainstay, along with grains, beans, and steamed vegetables (from the garden and the sea).

They also read Jason Winter's story of how he had cured himself. He had been a Hollywood stuntman who at the age of forty-six found out that he had "terminal" cancer—"infiltrating squamous cell carcinoma"—and was given just three months to live. Refusing to accept such a death sentence, he traveled the world in search of an herbal remedy. In the end he developed an herbal tea that sent his own cancer packing, and as a result, he began making it available to others. May added the now world-renowned Jason Winter's tea to her own battle plan.

Dietary supplements were also an important part of her self-directed program. Vitamin C, E, B-complex (to rid the body of excess estrogen), dietary fiber, flax seed oil, and more. Of course, there were also things to avoid. Red meat, white flour, sugar, caffeine—these were scratched from her menu, as were processed foods of any kind.

It's been eleven years now, and May's doing just fine. Six years ago she had to get a complete checkup before surgery for a jaw problem. At that time tests showed her free and clear of cancer. She hasn't been checked since. No need, as she sees it.

If she could do it over again, would she still have the surgery? "I don't think so," she answers. And the chemo? "To be honest, if I'd known then what I know now, I wouldn't have done even the few treatments that I did. I've just seen too many people die of cancer, who took conventional therapies all the way to their deaths."

Today May is leading health and cooking classes in her home, and she's working toward getting professionally trained as a licensed nutritional consultant. "I was a home economics major in college, and even taught it," she says, "but the nutrition I learned then is a whole lot different from what I've learned since getting cancer. We were taught a lot of the registered dietician kind of stuff— like white bread, jelly, and coffee were okay. That's not the kind of nutrition I want to teach. I just want to keep learning, to build up my knowledge and be able to help others. Ten years ago my doctors laughed at me. I don't really know where I got the courage or the conviction, but somehow I just knew that if I was going to get well, it was going to be through nutrition."

CHERYL WILKENS

Every cancer warrior has a personal story. Sometimes they tell of wonderful professionals who act as angels, gently guiding sick and hurting individuals along avenues of hope and healing. Other stories are more like a *Nightmare on Elm Street*. Scary, arrogant, self-absorbed doctors imposing their will, imprisoning their victims within the shackles of their own medical bigotry. Stories like that make us angry, make us distrust the medical community, make us want to do something to change things.

And then there are stories that seem to start down Elm Street, but through some brave action on the hero's part, end up at the intersection of help and renewed health. Cheryl Wilkens is just such a hero. And this is her story.

"My medical experiences opened my mind to alternative health care," she admits. "It all began three years ago when a tumor on the side of my knee and three moles on my back were removed. I was told by my surgeon that the tumor was merely fatty tissue, and the moles were all benign. In others words, he said these were nonmalignant conditions. Nothing to worry about.

"The following month, I showed him a lump that was growing back in the exact same area on my knee. 'It's just scar tissue,' he said with an arrogant brusqueness that told me he thought I was just a foolish woman. 'Go home, and don't worry about it.'"

Cheryl did as she was told, but four months later she was forced to return. The so-called "scar tissue" had grown. Not only that, it was hot. That got his attention. Another date with the knife was scheduled. Guess what, the lump that this doctor had disregarded as simply scar tissue was actually a serious malignancy.

"Immediately after the surgery, he told me that he was sure he'd gotten it all," recalls Cheryl. "However, the next day he called me at home to say that the lab work indicated that an even wider margin of tissue needed to be excised. I went back in and had it done later that week."

This third surgery really did a number on her leg. Only later was she fully informed as to the extent of what the surgeon had done. For now, all she knew was that it was badly disfigured, wouldn't work like it used to, and gave her constant pain.

"Again my surgeon told me that he was certain he had gotten it all, but he recommended that I have chemotherapy and radiation to eradicate any remaining cancer cells."

Wait a minute! Stop the story! Didn't he say he'd gotten it all the first time—the time before the lab informed him that he needed to do more? And if he thought he'd gotten it all this second time, why was he recommending chemo and radiation to kill remaining cancer cells? Could it be that the phrase "I think I got it all" simply has no meaning? Why don't doctors just tell it like it is: "I got the big stuff, but it's a guarantee that by the time a tumor is big enough to be felt, you'll have cancer cells roaming around unchecked all over in your body"?

And what about this doctor? Did he really know what he was

doing? Obviously not, for in talking with him later Cheryl found out that he'd done something entirely unacceptable in the world of medicine.

"I said to him that I couldn't understand why the first biopsy said the lump was benign, but when it grew back it was malignant. That's when he sort of made an off-the-cuff confession. Apparently, with the first lump he'd been so sure that it wasn't malignant that he hadn't even sent it to the lab."

Hadn't sent it to the lab! *Hadn't sent it to the lab!!* Who did this guy think he was—God? Friends told Cheryl she ought to sue his pants off. She and husband Larry considered it, but in the end decided to focus their energies on fighting cancer rather than medical malpractice. And although their trust in the surgeon's advice and character had been shattered (as well it should have been), they took the necessary steps to follow through on his suggestion of chemotherapy. It seemed their only option.

Cheryl soon found herself sitting in the office of a local oncologist. It was a Friday. "He opened my files for the first time and began to read through them. Without having previously studied them, he coolly recommended the maximum treatment of chemotherapy and radiation over the next six months. He assured me, however, that before anything was decided for sure, he would take some time over the weekend to check with other large institutions to see what they might recommend. I was to return to his office on Tuesday."

Tuesday rolled around. Cheryl kept her appointment, wondering what the oncologist had discovered. "I asked him what he'd learned from the other sources. He responded, 'Oh, I took my family skiing for three days and didn't have time to check it out.' Great! I then told him that I would be seeking a second opinion of my own. When he heard that, he abruptly stood up and walked out."

Cheryl and Larry did manage to get a second opinion. They eventually made their way to Mayo Clinic in Minnesota with medical records, pathology slides, and test results in hand. While there they learned news that further exploded even the smallest atoms of trust they might've still had floating around in their heads concerning their original surgeon.

"We took with us to Mayo the pathology slides of the moles I'd had removed the previous July and supposedly analyzed in Colorado Springs. Mayo's report concluded that they were 'a superficial spreading of level-3 melanoma.' The report my surgeon had given me, however, said 'no evidence of malignant melanoma.'"

Anyway, Cheryl also learned from the folks at Mayo things about conventional therapy that her potential oncologist had failed to tell her. She hadn't been warned that chemotherapy can permanently damage the kidneys, heart, and gall bladder. She had also not been informed that two of the four chemo drugs to be used were little more than experimental. It was an eye-opening trip to say the least!

Home again, Cheryl began looking into alternative therapies. She located Dr. Nicholas Gonzalez in New York City who had established a good reputation within the circles of alternative cancer treatments. His was a program of detoxification, nutrition, and supplements to help restore the body's immune system and innate ability to fight off cancer for itself. It was a protocol that had been originated over a twenty-five-year period by Dr. William Kelley, a dentist by training, who had become interested in helping people with chronic and degenerative disease. Gonzalez, a graduate of Cornell University Medical School, had conducted a five-year, 500-page case study of Kelley's patients while completing his training in immunology.

Although the Gonzalez staff carefully screens potential patients, turning down many they believe their protocol can't help, Cheryl was accepted. In the midst of preparing to leave for New York, her local surgeon asked her to come see him.

"He wanted to 'warn' me. He said that I had been the topic of conversation among fifteen of the top cancer specialists that morning, and that none of them had heard of the therapy I was investigating. He wanted me to know that I shouldn't waste my money on a 'quack' in New York. The look he then gave me would have crushed the hopes of any other patient. When he saw that I wasn't convinced, he looked uncomfortable, lost his posture, and said he needed to tell me what he had learned that day. He pulled a report from a file on his desk, and told me he had requested some information from the National Cancer Institute. The report said, 'The role of adjuvant chemotherapy in this setting is not fully defined and remains to be determined.' In other words, the effectiveness of chemotherapy on melanoma was unknown. No one really knew if it helped."

Although he had begun by spouting the "party line," her doctor was admitting that conventional therapy offered dubious hope. It made no sense to pursue a form of treatment that had no track record of working and, at the same time, would surely cause significant damage to her body. Off she and Larry went to the Big Apple.

"The results of blood work and hair analyses indicated that I had a great deal of cancer, with most of it probably throughout my lymphatic system," Cheryl recalls. "Dr. Gonzalez armed me with a vigorous metabolic program, no drugs."

The Kelley program classifies individuals by metabolic types— from slow-oxidizing vegetarians at one extreme to fast oxidizing carnivores at the other. Each person is unique, not only in nutritional needs but in food utilization as well. For each of the ten metabolic types, an individualized program is recommended.

There are, however, common threads that run through each. For instance, reduced protein intake accompanied by increased consumption of organic fruits and vegetables (including freshly made juices) is a central theme. During digestion, protein puts a strain on the body's enzyme force. This same enzyme force is a key player in fighting cancer cells. Reducing protein intake conserves enzyme power, enhancing their protective role in the body. (See *A Cancer Battle Plan*, page 71.)

The use of dietary supplements is also common to each personalized program. "Although getting all our nutrients from food should be our goal," says Cheryl, "the reality is that the body draws on stored vitamins and minerals when it doesn't get them from the foods we eat."

It's an unfortunate reality that modern farming techniques have robbed the soil, and thus the food chain, of many of the nutrients that used to be there. Daily megadoses of vitamins, minerals, and pancreatic enzymes help supply what the body needs to achieve reconstruction and well-being.

Finally, to assist with the process of detoxification, Gonzalez' patients use at least one coffee enema a day to help clean out the liver and gall bladder of toxins produced during tumor breakdown. The caffeine is absorbed into the bloodstream, delivered to the liver, and stimulates the liver and gallbladder to contract vigorously and dump bile, thus helping to clean them.

Cheryl has been battling against cancer for over two years now, and she's winning. Her cancer count, which began at thirty-five, is now down to seven. According to the scale Gonzalez uses, zero to five means cancer-free. Her ride through the rough waters of modern-day medical practice has left her with a lot to say.

Perhaps first on her list would be a warning to be fully informed before consenting to any surgery. "I knew my knee wasn't working the way it should. Sometime later, I read my surgeon's report for the first time and learned why. The patella tendon had been removed during the final surgery when the wider margin was removed. The surgeon had not told me this. No wonder my leg still won't pull me up a stairway. I asked my husband about this, and he said that after the operation, the surgeon told him he was able to save the leg. Save the leg?! He'd never said anything about the possibility of removing my tendon, much less my whole leg! If I could do it all over again, if I'd had surgery at all, I certainly wouldn't have consented to the last one that did so much damage."

Cheryl also has some pretty strong feelings about conventional cancer therapies. "Cutting, burning, and poisoning may help for a time, but they don't get to the cause of the disease. Many people are drug-oriented; we look for a single drug to cure or control a condition. We seek a quick fix by treating the symptoms, not the causes. My fundamental view is that to cure a disease like cancer, the conditions that caused it must be changed. If you don't go back to the imbalance in the body chemistry, to the weaknesses in the immune defenses, to whatever allowed the body to produce abnormal cells in the first place and correct things there, the likelihood is great that you will meet with this disease down the road again. It is imperative that we become nutritionally educated."

As concerns her choice to go with an alternative therapy as

the foundation of her cancer battle plan, Cheryl has this to say: "When you are diagnosed with cancer, you are introduced to yourself. You find out what you are made of. And when you choose alternative therapy, you find yourself living in a glass house. There will be people who will disagree with your choice. You have to stick with what you believe is best for you. Had I accepted the advice of my surgeon or oncologist, I very well could have been just another cancer statistic. I took the attitude of the Chinese proverb: 'Man who says it will not work, shouldn't disturb man who's making it work.' Until God opens another door, this alternative treatment is the best treatment for me."

Author's Notes

First, Cheryl had the unfortunate experience of working with a couple of doctors who didn't seem to have her best interests at heart. Please don't hear this story to say that either Cheryl or the authors think that all doctors are jerks or inept. The very fact that we quote M.D.'s throughout this book, plus writing about others, should be proof enough that we believe hundreds, if not thousands, of doctors are worthy of respect. Respect, of course, is not a gift. It must be earned.

Second, Cheryl and the thousands of other cancer warriors Anne and I have heard from as a result of our book *A Cancer Battle Plan* feel very strongly (as do growing numbers of M.D.'s and other medical professionals) about the inadequacy of a cancer-fighting strategy that includes only surgery, radiation, and/or chemotherapy. Cancer grows when the immune system has been compromised—either an inherited compromise passed from mother to child, or a developed compromise acquired over a number of years from diet, lifestyle, and environmental exposures. Surgery, radiation, and chemotherapy do nothing to rebuild the immune system. Their use in the cancer-fighting culture is akin to a wolf chewing off its leg to escape a trap. He's free, but he's got to do something about that wound if he's to survive long-term.

Sure, there are people (we can all probably name some) who were told nothing about the importance of rebuilding their immune systems following traditional cancer treatments, yet lived for years without recurrence. Is their experience the model to follow or promote? We think not. Every day here at *Health*Quarters, we hear from countless numbers of frustrated people for whom cancer is a recurrent visitor. "Why didn't anybody tell me about rebuilding my immune system ten years ago when I had that tumor removed?" "The chemo put my cancer into remission, but the doctors told me nothing about nutrition and rebuilding my immune system. They just said go home and enjoy life. That was three years ago. Now my cancer's back."

Cheryl has discovered, as have thousands of others, that the use of surgery, radiation, and chemotherapy in battling cancer is a matter of treating the symptoms not the causes. They may be important allies in the overall war, but the best chance for long-term victory lies in rebuilding the body's God-given army of defense, the immune system.

TOM MCKINNEY
"I hate the damn stuff!"

If you ask Tom McKinney's opinion about carrot juice, he doesn't pull any punches. It's not his cup of tea. At the same time, he has come to recognize and appreciate the powerful punch of nutrients that carrots deliver—things like beta-carotene, vitamin B-complex, vitamins C, D, E, K, iron, calcium, phosphorus, sodium, potassium, magnesium, manganese, sulphur, and copper. And juicing carrots multiplies their "pow."

"When you drink a glass of carrot juice," Tom explains, "you've taken in the equivalent of an awful lot of carrots."

Tom's initiation into the world of juice came in the early years of his seventh decade. Right about the time he turned seventy he started to have problems with his prostate. "You've certainly got a prostate problem," agreed his urologist as he looked at test results. "Unfortunately, you also have colon cancer."

Colon cancer? Oh no! And before dealing with his prostate, his doctors insisted that they first operate on his colon. In all, they removed fourteen inches. In the process, they discovered that the cancer had migrated.

"Not only was it in my colon and prostate, but it had spread to my gallbladder and pelvic bone." After informing him that he had two months to live, his doctors set about the process of trying to prolong his days by poisoning his system. "They gave me some chemo that made me vomit around the clock. I was heaving so hard that I ruptured my groin area. They repaired the hernia, but it cost me an extra seven days in the hospital. Not only that, but the chemo didn't affect my cancer at all. All that throwing up for nothing."

Hernia patched, his doctors wanted to dive back in after his prostate, taking his testicles as well. "But by that time," recalls Tom, "my wife and I had been reading a lot of books and talking with people around the country. We said, 'No way,' and decided to go the naturopathic route."

Managing to get himself out of that hospital bed before he lost more of his irreplaceables, Tom was soon off to see a local naturopathic doctor who had reportedly helped a lot of people. "When she first examined me, I'd just come home from the colon surgery. She didn't know anything about me, other than my name. She used iridology, saliva tests, and reflexology to tell me everything that was happening with my body. She was accurate to the 'nth' degree. In fact, she told me more in thirty minutes about my health problems than the M.D.'s had in two years."

The next fourteen months found Tom devoted to a nutritional battle plan against the cancer that had taken over his midsection. The whole point of the therapy was to treat the body, not the disease. In other words, repair and rebuild the functioning of his immune system and various organs so that cancer could not survive. His liver, pancreas, and kidneys were in bad shape and needed a lot of help.

The diet he was to follow required that he avoid red meat, in fact all meat for at least the first four months. Also to be avoided were white flour, sugar, and dairy products of all kinds. Raw, organic fruits and vegetables became the focus, plus lots and lots of freshly squeezed juices. In addition, he was to take a daily smorgasbord of dietary supplements meant to further enhance the quality and quantity of nutrients with which his body could reconstruct health.

Today at seventy-five years of age, Tom McKinney still hates carrot juice. But he loves the fact that—except for fourteen inches of large intestine—he's still all here and his cancer is still all gone.

"I can't say enough good things about what my naturopathic doctor and her diet did for me," he says gushing with gratitude. "I got up off my deathbed, and I feel like a million dollars!"

JUNE PRUITT

June Pruitt lay on the sofa in her living room, fighting off nausea as she tried to give direction to the daily activities of her three children. Because her husband traveled so much in his job, their twelve-year-old son had been pressed into the role of "chief cook and dish washer" for himself and two younger brothers. She couldn't help wondering if she'd ever get better. Her life had taken on the desperate emotions of someone trapped in a personal prison from which there was no escape. "Life for me had become a real nightmare," she recalls.

It all began one day when Jane came face to face with what was considered certain death. The doctors called it multiple myeloma. "It's considered a fatal form of cancer," she explains, "which causes bones to develop lesions, creating honeycomb effects that can fracture when a person is touched or picked up."

In the months that followed her diagnosis, June was subjected to enough toxic drugs to float a battleship. However, none worked to turn the tide in her favor, as her health and spirits drifted slowly out to sea. "I felt totally destroyed, both mentally and physically. Just being alive had become a heavy burden. My hair fell out, my immune system crashed, I got a lung infection, and finally my lungs collapsed. I was close to death. The doctors told us that I could not tolerate any more chemotherapy and that it would be best to just try to keep me comfortable with painkillers until I died."

If there was a bottom to hit, she'd hit it. What life she had left was to be lived out on a sofa. It's not hard to imagine the level of despair she must have felt as she watched the world go by without her active involvement. Questions, no doubt, haunted her. What would her husband do once she was gone? Would he remarry? And what about the kids? How would they take her death? What would they be like when they grew up? Who would they marry? What would their kids be like?

During this time, while she was waiting around to die, June began to hear reports about alternative therapies for cancer. People were being helped, even after the medical community had given up on them. A spark of hope was rekindled. But she would have to travel. "I realized that the clinics doing these sorts of things were not in the U.S. and that I would have to leave the country to get the kind of help I was looking for." That's just what she did.

The particular clinic June eventually decided on was in Jamaica. Its doors are no longer open, although similar therapies are still done in Mexico.[2] June describes her experience this way: "My therapy consisted of fresh juices, fruits and vegetables, and a nontoxic treatment that included proteolytic enzymes in conjunction with vitamin B_{17}, also known as Laetrile. I was given high doses of water-soluble vitamin A to help rebuild my immune system. The staff were all licensed doctors and registered nurses, the environment was upbeat and stress-free, and the cost was extremely low compared to what my insurance company had paid for the toxic therapies back in the U.S. Of course, my insurance refused to pay for the treatment I received in Jamaica since it didn't meet the procedures set forth by the American Medical Association, but it was worth paying for it myself. It was making me well."

So *well* did she get that she found herself up to taking on another fight. She joined a group of people who went to court in Florida to try to win back freedom of choice for cancer patients in the kinds of therapies they wished to pursue. They ultimately lost the Laetrile issue to the overbearing political muscle of the AMA and FDA, but they gave it their best shot.

"I don't advocate that Laetrile treatment works for everyone, although I know it has been a part of my own success," she says. "I am convinced that the individual must have the right to choose whatever sort of therapies are right for him and he's comfortable with. Because we don't have that freedom of choice in the U.S., we have lost some of our civil rights."

Nonetheless, June is still alive and kicking. She has taken

charge of her own health and, with the help of her family, maintains a diet and lifestyle aimed at keeping cancer from returning. "I undergo 'live cell therapy' to enhance my immune system. We eat a diet rich in fresh fruits, vegetables, beans, sprouted seeds, and fish. We drink distilled water. And I regularly use coffee enemas to keep my system free of toxic buildup. I thank God for my returned health and loving family who were at my side through this catastrophic ordeal."

Having come back from the "near dead," obviously June also feels a strong pull—more than the average person might—toward making an impact on her world with whatever life she has left. She intends to keep at the cause that has captured her attention and energized her soul into action. "Good health prevailing," she promises, "I will continue to fight for patients' rights in health care."

MARIJAMAH MIRIAM VERNON

Australian Marijamah Miriam Vernon hit what she thought was just a small bump, a temporary annoyance, along the road through life. A suspicious-looking mole on her left leg was removed for laboratory tests. The results—malignant melanoma, stage 4. In other words, it was cancer, and it had spread. An operation followed to remove a large amount of tissue from the surrounding area. "And I thought that would be the end of it. I knew nothing about melanoma and what might happen to me down the road."

Something did happen. Three years later a large tumor was found settled into her left groin area. The cancer had been at work. "My specialist wanted to book me for surgery immediately," she recalls. "Stunned, I needed time to think through my situation. I was being told that even with surgery and chemotherapy, I could expect at best to live only a handful of years."

She and her husband began to read up on cancer and alternative therapies. One book that impressed them was Dr. Max Gerson's *A Cancer Therapy* in which he outlined the therapy he used for years with terminal cancer patients, along with the results from fifty cases. In simple terms, Gerson believed in cleaning and detoxifying the liver, the key organ in the body for battling cancer. He also believed in the necessity of restoring the body's innate ability to protect itself, by rebuilding the immune system. Both, he contended, could be accomplished through diet and related nontoxic therapies. Juice fasting and coffee enemas to stimulate the liver to dump bile and thus clean itself were examples of such therapies.

"A very strong impression came over me," Marijamah recalls, "that I had to take personal responsibility for what I had done to my health. I decided that never again would I put my life in someone else's hands or allow my body to be cut up every time another tumor appeared."

With her husband's full support, the next day she launched herself in the direction of a full and intensive cleansing and dietary program built upon Max Gerson's advice. "It was scary," she admits. "But at the same time I had a great feeling of peace and calm."

To say that it was hard would be an understatement. The lady from "down under" had her life turned "upside down." The Gerson therapy is not something a person can do on the backstroke or add to an otherwise crammed calendar. It becomes a full-time job, the work of getting well. It requires, in fact, it demands center stage. There are juices to be made and consumed every hour of the day. There are enemas to be undertaken regularly each day. And there is a special diet to be prepared. It takes discipline, not only time-wise but attitude-wise as well. Change is hard, especially when it comes to changing one's diet. From this reporter's experience, it seems that people might more easily change their religion than change their diet. Of all things that people cling to most ferociously, it's the food they draw comfort and pleasure from.

Marijamah was willing to make the necessary changes. Her life, you see, was at stake. She gave it everything she had. "From day one," she says, "I stuck with it 100 percent. Seven days a week, twenty-four hours a day. Looking back, that was the key to my success—100 percent commitment."

Looking after herself, something she'd never been all that good about, was a real challenge. To keep herself motivated and moving forward, Marijamah approached the whole thing as a project—a fascinating journey toward health and healing on all levels.

"Our kitchen became filled with fresh, live organic food. My heart would fill with joy whenever my husband came home from shopping laden with boxes of living foods, organically grown the way nature designed foods to grow, filled with balanced nutrients and enzymes. I learned to value and have respect for the fresh foods I ate and juiced. Flooding oneself intensively every day with the live enzymes in these foods, one's body simply can't help but turn from dying to becoming alive. And that's exactly what happened to me. My tumor dissolved, and I could feel my health turning around. I started putting on needed weight. And I went from a grayish tint to a healthy glow. Seeing the pollution that came from my body, along with the dead cancer, was a bit of a miracle."

As was said, this was not an easy process. There were hard times, both physically and emotionally. But she stayed with it for two solid years, monitored all the while by a caring doctor who kept track of her progress. After a year she went back to see the original specialist who had told her that surgery was her only option. He was duly impressed by her progress. In fact, after the second year he gave her a clean bill of health. "We're proud of you," he said, and sent a report to the Gerson clinic in Mexico concerning her recovery.

Now, several years after the discovery of the tumor in her groin, Marijamah Miriam Vernon has this to say about what she's learned about health and healing: "Physical healing starts from within. Our bodies can heal themselves on all levels, given the right environment, love, support, and faith in our Creator. I am enjoying a healthy life, keeping to this live-foods diet. As Dr. Gerson said in his book, 'Stay close to nature, and its eternal laws will protect you.'"

DORIS HENDERSON
Sometimes patients fall through the cracks of the modern health-care system. Busy doctors, faced with the growing onslaught of degenerative disease, can sometimes forget about commitments and promises they've made to various individual patients as they hurry around trying to fulfill all their obligations. Hey, they're only human.

For the unfortunate patient who has become one of the "forgotten"—overlooked or simply lost in the shuffle—it can be devastating, both physically and emotionally. Even so, there are folks like Doris Henderson who have found ways and means of turning into blessing being lost in the medical maze.

Five years ago, Doris discovered a lump in her breast. "It was just a small lump," she explains. "I had a lumpectomy and radiation, and the doctors told me there was less than a 1 percent chance that it would return. Well, guess what."

About a year ago, Doris noticed a feeling of weakness in her left hip. Her doctor, thinking it bursitis, sent her to physical therapy. When that didn't clear it up, an orthopedic surgeon was consulted. His X-ray showed a shadow. A biopsy confirmed her fear. *It's baaaack.* And a total-body bone scan revealed the ugly truth. It wasn't just back, but all over the place—spine, pelvic bone, skull, shoulders. "Every place but my arms and legs," recalls Doris.

"Time for chemo," said her oncologist, putting her on Tamoxifin. Over the next months, the cancer got no worse, but neither did it get better. Bone density tests revealed that the disease had eaten a good deal of the hip. A surgical hip replacement was performed, followed a few months later by another bone scan.

"That's when my doctor suggested the bone marrow transplant (BMT)," recalls Doris. "The cancer just wasn't responding to the Tamoxifin. He figured the BMT was my best bet and told me he'd get a hold of those people to call me."

And that's when Doris fell through the proverbial crack. She never did hear back from either him or them. "I think he just forgot about me," she says of her oncologist. "I really did want to explore the transplant option. I do think it's important to educate yourself on all possibilities. But they forgot me."

For Doris, exploring her options meant reading everything she could get her hands on. Her sister handed her a book that totally redirected her battle efforts. It was *A Cancer Battle Plan*, by yours truly.

"By the time I realized I wasn't going to hear from those people, I'd already started seeing a nutritionist and was well into a nutritional program that I wanted to stay with anyway," Doris admits.

So, has it helped?

"Oh, yes, very much so! I went back for another bone scan recently, the first one since going on the nutritional program. It showed much improvement. The radiologist made marks all over it where healing was obvious. Some of the spots that had been there are gone. Others are fading or smaller."

So, Doris, what does your nutritional program consist of?

"Well, it's very similar to what's outlined in *A Cancer Battle Plan*. Fasting at first with freshly made juices, along with enemas every day to clean the colon and the liver. That's followed by a vegetarian diet that is strong on raw, organic fruits and vegetables. Plus, I take lots of supplements that have been specifically matched to what my blood work shows my body needs."

What would you say to others fighting cancer?

"I'd tell them that nutrition is certainly worth a try. It seems to be working for me. I'm not against a bone marrow transplant, but I'd rather try this way first."

Author's Note

Every day, here at *Health*Quarters, we get calls and letters from people all over the U.S. who are fighting cancer. Many have had bone marrow transplants, only to have the disease return within months or a very few years. Unfortunately, most were never informed that simply killing cancer cells, the focus of the BMT and related chemo, is not enough. The ultimate goal in winning against cancer is to create an environment in the body where cancer cannot grow. That can be accomplished only by restoring to power the body's own army of health soldiers, the God-given immune system.

That doesn't just happen. It takes work, a lot of work. Everything you eat or drink, the quality of air you breathe, even the stresses you're under, can have an impact on the health of your immune system. The fact that you have cancer in the first place is a sign that your immune system has somehow already been compromised by your diet, lifestyle, and/or environment. Chemo, radiation, surgery, and even a bone marrow transplant (which, by the way, includes massive doses of chemo) serve to further wound the immune system, although in some instances they may be a viable first step toward fighting back.

It's much like a wolf chewing off his leg to escape from a trap. He will need to do much, much more if he hopes to survive very long. So, too, the cancer patient who selects the BMT or any of the other invasive therapies. As we've said, rebuilding the immune system is the only way to create an environment where cancer can't live.

So if you're exploring the possibility of a bone marrow transplant to help in your own battle plan against cancer, please do remember that whatever weapons you initially incorporate, ultimately you will need to use those that serve to rebuild your immune system.

REV. GEORGE MALKMUS

The good Reverend Malkmus, up until recently, ran a health-food store and restaurant in a small town in Tennessee. Problem was, it got too successful. "It grew so fast," he says, "that it required almost total commitment of my time, eight-plus hours a day, six days a week."

At the same time, the health-oriented ministry, which he founded and dubbed Hallelujah Acres (of which the store and restaurant were just a part), was being overwhelmed by requests for seminars, public appearances, and literature. The decision was made to give up the store and restaurant and to concentrate his efforts on impacting a wider audience. Even just keeping up with publishing and sending out his newsletter, *Back to the Garden*, had become a challenge. Issue 1 came out in May of 1993 and was sent to 4,000 subscribers. Issue 6 (January/February 1994) had an initial printing of 12,000, and they had to reprint 4,000 more!

Intrigued by this interesting man and his unique vision, I gave him a call one day not long ago.

DAVE: "I'm intrigued and excited by your ministry of health. How did you get involved in nutrition?"

REV. MALKMUS: "Eighteen years ago, I lost my mother to colon cancer. She was a nurse and went the traditional

medical route with very devastating results. It was
clear to me that the treatment, not the cancer, caused
her death. I was forty-two at the time. Believe it or not,
shortly after my mother's death, I was diagnosed with
colon cancer myself. I had a tumor the size of a base-
ball. I didn't know anything about nutritional therapies
at that point, but I knew I wasn't going to let the doctors do to me what I'd just seen them do to my
mother."

DAVE: "Let's see, that would make you sixty years old
now. You sound pretty healthy for a guy with a base-
ball-sized tumor in his colon. What did you do to help
yourself?"

REV. MALKMUS: "First of all, I refused any invasive
medical treatment. I was persuaded by a friend to
change my diet to only raw foods, with lots of carrot
juice. Overnight, I switched. In fact, I didn't eat a
single piece of cooked food for over a year."

DAVE: "Did it do any good?"

REV. MALKMUS: "Better than that. Every physical problem
I'd had, not just the tumor, was gone in less than a
year. No more hypoglycemia, no more hemorrhoids,
no more allergies, no more sinus problems, no more
high blood pressure, and no more to a bunch of other
little things. For the last eighteen years I have not
experienced so much as a cold, sore throat, headache,
upset stomach, been to a doctor, or taken so much as
an aspirin. I'm sixty years old and can still play foot-
ball and basketball with the boys, jog five miles a day,
and do more than most teenagers can."

DAVE: "That's incredible! Have others had similar success
with a raw foods diet?"

REV. MALKMUS: "Oh, yes! We're seeing friends who are
diagnosed with terminal cancer get going on such a
diet. Six months later, the doctors can't find cancer.
People with diabetes, two weeks to four months later,
are off insulin and their blood sugar level is normal.

We've seen folks with arthritis become pain-free in thirty days. In an upcoming issue of our newsletter we're featuring the story of a woman who came to us a little over a year ago weighing 275 pounds and suffering from rheumatoid arthritis. She couldn't get out of bed alone. Her husband had to dress her, brush her teeth, and comb her hair. The doctors said she'd soon be in a wheelchair. Just a year after changing her diet, she's lost 112 pounds and her arthritis is gone. It's just incredible the body God has given each of us. We know that our automobiles won't run right if we use the wrong kind of fuel. The same is true about our bodies."

DAVE: "Any negative feedback from the medical community?"

REV. MALKMUS: "We actually have a lot of doctors coming to our seminars and going on our program. A doctor was here recently from Wisconsin. He flew all the way here just to attend one of my seminars. He's going back to put into practice what we teach. It's incredible the number of doctors who are excited about the natural approach to health and healing—and I'm talking about M.D.'s. They're realizing that what they've got doesn't work, that what they're doing is actually making people worse."

QUOTES

"After visiting a wholistic health care clinic . . . I became especially impressed with the effectiveness of raw food diets and natural remedies used during the treatment of patients with disorders ranging from cancer and mental health problems, to multiple sclerosis."

—Robert Buist, Ph.D., D.O.
TOWNSEND LETTER FOR DOCTORS

"Our cancer research is misdirected, inefficient, and inadequate. We have almost as many people living off the disease as

are dying from it. The government spends billions on cancer research, but at the same time allows known carcinogens in our processed foods, subsidizes cigarettes, and continues to develop new radiation, surgical, and chemotherapy techniques when burning, cutting, and poisoning have already proved largely unsuccessful. Physicians have not been trained in preventive medicine and, not having experience or knowledge of preventive medicine, they continue the outmoded but orthodox approach of treating symptoms rather than the entire body. . . . Many doctors today are committed in their mind to the straitjacket placed on them by their medical training. . . . Often it is the nurse who sees the patient and ends up having more time with the cancer victim than the attending physician. What a world of good the nurses could accomplish if they were better informed about the nutritional way to combat disease, about the metabolic processes, and about the need for therapeutic augmentation of concentrated nutrients—vitamins and minerals."

—Richard O. Brennan, M.D., D.O.
Coronary? Cancer? God's Answer: Prevent It!

"America is a consumer driven society. It is you who will create the momentum for change. Don't wait for some government organization, or new law, or general endorsement from one of the major health care organizations to implement nutrition as part of a comprehensive cancer treatment. It has been said that all truth must go through three stages: first, it is rejected; second, it is violently opposed; third, it is accepted as self-evident. Nutrition in cancer treatment currently resides on stage two, and is moving swiftly toward stage three. When is the evidence enough? Right now!"

—Patrick Quillin, Ph.D., R.D.
Beating Cancer With Nutrition

FURTHER READING
Beating Cancer With Nutrition by Patrick Quillin Ph.D., R.D., with Noreen Quillin (Tulsa, OK: The Nutrition Times Press, Inc., 1994).

A Cancer Battle Plan by Anne Frähm with David Frähm (Colorado Springs, CO: Piñon Press, 1992).

A Cancer Therapy by Max Gerson, M.D. (Bonita, CA: The Gerson Institute in association with Station Hill Press, Inc., New York; 5th edition, 1990).

Crackdown on Cancer With Good Nutrition by Ruth Yale Long, Ph.D. (Houston, TX: Nutrition Education Association, Inc., 1989).

Nutrition, The Cancer Answer by Maureen Salaman (Menlo Park, CA: Statford Publishing, 1984).

NOTES
1. Albert Schweitzer, as quoted in *A Cancer Therapy* (Results of Fifty Cases) by Max Gerson, M.D. (Bonita, CA: The Gerson Institute, 1990), Book Cover.
2. Many Mexican clinics are highly regarded within alternative therapy circles. Ignorance, however, breeds contempt. Most Americans lack information concerning alternative cancer-treatment centers outside the familiar boundaries of the USA, the AMA, and the FDA. This leaves us with a mental picture of a bunch of unqualified quacks dispensing bogus potions while they suck the life savings right out of their patients' bank accounts.

6

NUTRITION AND CANDIDA

INTRODUCTION TO CANDIDA

Most people have some knowledge about the majority of health problems represented in this book. For instance, when we say allergies or cancer or diabetes, some sort of mental picture probably comes to your mind that helps you define and relate to what we're talking about. Perhaps your definition lacks a full understanding of the complexity of the ailment, but it gives you a reference point, nonetheless.

But what comes to your mind when you read the title to this chapter? Nothing? You're not alone. Most people know nothing about *candida*, yet all of us have it. And if we're not careful it can have its way with us, reaping all kinds of havoc upon our health.

John Trowbridge, M.D., is a leading authority on candida. Here's his definition:

Candida albicans (full name) is a yeast growth present in and on most of us which is normally controlled by our immune defenses and by the usual bacterial flora present in and on the body. But when an ecological change takes place in the internal environment, helpful bacteria tend to be decreased and immune response becomes depressed.

Then the yeast begins to increase in the body, especially in the colon (large intestine). These yeast colonies release powerful chemicals (toxins) that may be absorbed into the bloodstream, causing such widely varying symptoms as severe menstrual cramps in women and lethargy, chronic diarrhea, bladder irritations and infections, asthma, migraine headaches, depression, skin eruptions, and many other difficulties in both men and women. Localized areas of Candida overgrowth cause other obvious, recurrent and persistent infections such as yeast vaginitis, oral thrush, and rashes. These problems often herald the insidious beginning of the deeper-seated and more dangerous inner infections. Thus, a myriad of symptoms and signs are the Candida-caused human disorders collectively referred to as "candidiasis."

Fifty years ago doctors identified *Candida albicans* as a frequent cause of vaginal, mouth, throat, and gastrointestinal tract infections. Now it's well known to affect almost all body parts, organs, tissues, and cells. Research physicians suspect Candida as a complication in AIDS, a contributor to early death in various forms of cancer, a source of infertility in some women, and a mischief-maker in other medical tragedies such as MS, myasthenia gravis, schizophrenia, and arthritis.[1]

The sort of yeast overgrowth that Trowbridge is talking about can be caused by a handful of agents that we purposefully (albeit, ignorantly) allow into our bodies. These include birth control pills, steroid-related drugs like cortisone and prednisone, and antibiotics. Even the antibiotics in the animal products we consume can kill the yeast police (the healthy bacteria) in our bodies.

The following stories tell how three people rebuilt that yeast police force in their bodies.

DIANE HAWKINS

"You know that stuff that you use to strip paint off furniture— the stuff that really burns when you get it on your hands? That's how the pain in my vagina felt. It was horrible! Real agony! I'd have to put ice between my legs at night just to relieve the pain enough so I could get some sleep."

For Diane Hawkins, life had become a miserable trudge from one doctor to the next. Although she and her husband made their home in what many people might consider paradise—the island of Bermuda where he worked for the U.S. government—her life had become a living hell.

"Ever since my son was born," recalls Diane, "more and more often I kept getting urinary tract infections. I'd drink cranberry juice and take vitamin C. Eventually the infection would go away."

But there came a point when the infection decided to put in for resident status. No matter what she tried on her own, she couldn't shake it. The military doctors on base were consulted. Finding nothing wrong, other than a little bacteria in her urine, antibiotic medication was prescribed in hopes that it would clear up whatever mysterious infection was hiding in her urinary tract. Bad decision. Urinary tract infections, also known as bladder infections, are bacterial and respond to antibiotics. However, antibiotics don't kill yeast, which is a fungus. And yeast overgrowth was exactly what was happening in Diane's body, starting in her vagina.

Actually, antibiotics do only one thing for yeast. They make it worse. They kill off the good bacteria as well as the bad. It's the good bacteria that keeps the naturally occurring yeast in our bodies in check. Antibiotics are to yeast what gasoline is to fire. The stage had been set for a full-blown, guns-drawn, five-alarm yeast takeover, otherwise known as *candida*.

Only antifungal products will work to combat yeast. (Some of these are mentioned in the books listed at the end of this chapter on page 122.) They include things like Nystatin, Nizoral, Diflucan, Fungistatin, lactobacillus acidophilus, caprylic acid, Tanalbit, citrus seed and extracts, and garlic products, including Kyolic. In fact, if you check the topical creams sold these days to women for vaginal yeast overgrowth, you'll note that they are labeled antifungal, not antibiotic.

"I'd lie in bed with this terrible pain in my abdomen. None

of the doctors could tell me what it was. They could never find anything. I was afraid I had some kind of cancer and was going to die."

Meanwhile, her doctors continued to test urine samples and prescribe antibiotics, never thinking they ought to do a vaginal check. This, by the way, was a significant oversight. Women with the type of complaint Diane was bringing are normally and routinely checked for yeast overgrowth, an easily diagnosed condition.

"It took a full year and a half to finally get this stuff diagnosed correctly. The urine tests they kept taking would come back normal every time. It got to the point where the doctors began looking at me as if the pain was all in my head—psychosomatic. They had run every test in the book, or so they thought. They even tested me for all sorts of sexually transmitted diseases. It was very humiliating and horrible."

A batch of new doctors were assigned to the base. Unfortunately, they sang the same old tired tune—"We just don't see anything wrong with you . . . blah, blah, blah, blah, blah."

But things were just about to change for the better. A magazine came into her hands suggesting that sometimes the very best place to get medical advice is from the public health services. Off she went to search for a new source of help, someone who could answer the question, "What's wrong with me?"

The nurse put me up on the table and did a vaginal swab. "Diane," she said, "you're absolutely crawling with yeast!" Finally, somebody who could label the source of her mysterious pain! It was as if a dark cloud that had hung close overhead had suddenly been lifted. Her fears of cancer vanished, the sun came out, birds sang, and hope once again filled her heart. Now the question was, "How do you fight off yeast?"

"The nurse got me headed in the right direction. She was wonderful. I would go in to see her early in the morning before anyone else arrived. She put me on some medication that attacked the yeast. She also started me on the process of removing things from my diet that fed it. Dairy products were the first to go. Dairy causes mucus to be produced in the body. Yeast thrives on mucus."

Books—like *The Yeast Connection* by William Crook, M.D., and *Fit for Life* by Harvey and Marilyn Diamond—also guided her as she made her way toward better health and healing. They mentioned other kinds of foods she should avoid: things with yeast, sugar, vinegar, anything aged. Fruit and fruit juices can also be a problem, because these have so much naturally occurring sugar.

"I still have problems occasionally if I eat sugary things," she says. Stress also sets off the yeast. Her teenaged son is in a health battle of his own. The cancer she feared for herself reared its ugly head in her son's leg. A mother can't help but feel stress as she watches her child battle his way through a very dangerous disease. But he seems to be doing just fine these days. The health problems that have plagued the Hawkins family may be a thing of the past. They're working hard diet-wise to help keep it that way.

What would Diane say to others who are experiencing some of the same symptoms she had?

"First, if you're having repeated urinary problems, suspect candida." In other words, get yourself checked for yeast overgrowth. Don't just assume that it's an infection that antibiotics will handle. If your urinary problems are caused by yeast, antibiotics will make it worse. "Second, get off dairy products to see if that helps."

There's another thing in all this that begs to be said, and perhaps Diane hasn't said it because she doesn't want to ruffle too many feathers. We'll say it because it's very important—in fact, essential. It's this: Keep going until you get answers, answers that make sense to you. It's your body. You're the boss in your battle for health. Everyone else is just hired help. If you have pain, something's wrong. Don't let anybody dissuade you from getting the help you need just because their ability to read your symptoms is woefully inadequate or professionally biased. In the case of candida, some doctors just don't think it exists. You may find in your own war to win back your health that part of your fight is with medical ignorance and related arrogance. Hang in there. Keep at it until you find somebody who can adequately address your needs. Diane did, and for that she's to be applauded.

DAVE FRÄHM

I remember that long before I knew what was happening to me I'd lie awake nights with pain in my gut, as fears flooded my head that

I had colon cancer. I'd toss for hours, sinking deeper and deeper into a "blue funk," wondering what my wife and kids would do without me once I was dead. Sometimes I'd get up and use an enema for relief. Constipation seemed to hound me. Other times I'd start working at my computer. I just couldn't sleep—at least not long, or well.

Then morning would come. The Colorado sun would shine. I'd go out and walk a couple of brisk miles around the neighborhood, filling my lungs with fresh air. The depression would lift, my mood would change, and life would look hopeful once again.

So what was behind those tremendous mood swings? Why was I "down in the dumps" at night and sure I was dying of cancer, when each morning would find me "on top of the world" and doing just fine?

It all began when I contracted a severe chest cold that I couldn't shake through natural means. Perhaps I was just being impatient. Nevertheless, I went to a drop-in health clinic and got a prescription for some very strong antibiotic drugs to take over the next couple of weeks.

What I didn't know back then, that I know all too well now, is that anytime you take antibiotics, you should take certain things to help keep the naturally occurring yeast in your body from roaring out of control. You want to help kill off yeast, plus replace the good bacteria in the bowel that antibiotics disrupt and destroy.

Anyhow, shortly after finishing my couple of weeks on antibiotics I began to develop all the symptoms of a classic case of systemic yeast overgrowth, otherwise known as *candida albicans*—candida, for short. At the time I had no idea that all of these annoyances were related. My symptoms included:

▲ "Crotch rot" (itching and rash in the crotch area)
▲ Athlete's foot (itching and rash between the toes)
▲ A "clouded" toenail (white, not clear)
▲ Poor elimination and constipation, sometimes alternating with diarrhea
▲ Pain and gripping in lower part of colon
▲ Intense rectal itching

▲ Depression
▲ Insomnia
▲ "Short fuse" irritability
▲ Sensitivity to certain foods, which within a few hours lowered my energy level and brought on a sore throat
▲ Increased sensitivity to chemicals and other irritants in the air, which would drain my energy
▲ Unusually sore muscles in chest and back, plus tingling and numbness in left hand and arm

As I said, all this was happening to me before I realized that everything was connected to yeast overgrowth. I just figured that "crotch rot" was the end result of underwear that was too tight on body parts too moist. I had no idea that it was somehow connected to a cloudy toenail on my big toe (evidence that yeast had been at work). Nor did it occur to me that athlete's foot had any part in this puzzle. And only later did I learn that uncontrolled yeast releases chemicals into the bloodstream that affect brain chemistry, resulting often in depression, insomnia, and irritability. The fact that oxygen helps to kill off yeast explains why my early morning walks always seemed to get me "up" from "down."

Anyhow, after reading a book on candida, I finally began to see how all that I was experiencing fit together. That in itself—the ability to put a name to it all—boosted my spirits.

I went to a different doctor, this time one who knew the connection between antibiotics, candida, and nutritional issues. He prescribed an antifungal medication to help kill off yeast. (By the way, he concurred with my self-diagnosis that I, indeed, had a systemic yeast problem.) There are several yeast fighting drugs available. The most commonly recommended seems to be Nystatin, although I was prescribed Sporanox because it tends to get into the bloodstream better.

Besides the medication, I also began to take natural yeast killing products, as well as things to reestablish the good bacteria in my colon. There are many non-drug, nonprescription products on the market for controlling yeast. Raw garlic, for instance, is very effective. Garlic also comes in odorless forms. I used a product called Kyolic, produced by Waukunaga of America. Melaluca oil, also known as Australian tea tree oil, is another yeast-fighting product. Other weapons in my yeast fighting arsenal included Fungistatin made by Molecular and Yeast Fighters by Twin Labs.

To help restore the natural flora, there are also many products available. The kind I used most was Acidophilase, another of Waukunaga of America's products. What you're looking for here are products that contain acidophilus. That's the friendly bacteria that prevail in our intestine and keep harmful bacteria and yeast in check.

The biggest and hardest part of my battle plan, however, was and is the diet. Foods need to be avoided that feed yeast. A person with yeast problems should have no products with sugar, fructose, honey, molasses, maple syrup, or other related sweeteners. No products with yeast—that means breads, pastries, many cereals, and on and on (the grain product may also be feeding the yeast and causing the problem). No aged products or things with mold—that includes soy sauce, mushrooms, cheese, and vinegar. Oh, rats, not vinegar! Do you realize how many salad dressings, even natural ones, have vinegar in them?! Of course, most of them also have some sort of honey or sweetener. Double whammy! And finally, no fruits or fruit juices—at least for a while. The diet part of this fight has been hard.

Although I'm making progress, the hardest time for me is when I'm feeling better. I tend to want to eat something—oh, a piece of fruit or some spaghetti sauce—otherwise healthy but not good for fighting candida. When I do, my symptoms come roaring back. Candida is not usually something you work on for a day or a week and get rid of. It's not usually something that you can deal with on the backstroke. It often takes months, sometimes, years.

My current diet? At this point I am eating eggs, the kind produced by chickens that are fed organic feed and allowed to roam freely. I eat cereals that don't have any sugars, yeast, etc., in them. I've learned to read labels very carefully. Did you realize that Grape Nuts has yeast in it? We use Rice Dream at our house, a wonderfully tasty milk substitute made from, you guessed it, rice. In addition, raw or steamed veggies, brown rice, various grains and whole grain pastas, potatoes, soups, and salads round out what I eat.

If I were you, I'd think twice and thrice about ever using antibiotics. If you really need them, okay. But make sure you work hard at keeping the balance in your system. You also need to know that birth control pills and steroids can bring on candida. So can eating meat. Most livestock these days are given large doses of antibiotics. It's a package deal. You eat the animal, you get the drugs.

If you're experiencing any of the symptoms you find in these stories, you ought to pick up one of the excellent titles that follow (see page 122), and do some self-diagnosing. If you have a yeast problem, better to get after it now than to wait until after it has time to really reap havoc.

DEBBIE LOUTHAN

She was just twenty-two years old—a time in life for spreading one's wings, charting a new course, and venturing out into the big world to see what life and living is really all about. For most, twenty-two is an age of innocence, a time relatively free from the cares and concerns that come with each additional candle added to the birthday cake. But for this young woman, something was wrong. Something was driving her inward and downward. Something was stealing her passion for life and her reason for living.

"To be honest with you," says Debbie Louthan, now twenty-six, "I was thinking suicide. Not to the point where I would've actually done it, but I was severely depressed. *Why keep on living, I thought to myself, if life is going to be like this?*"

Indeed, something awful was happening to Debbie. Her body seemed to be coming apart at the seams. She was besieged by chronic fatigue, chronic indigestion, chronic headaches, chronic muscle pains, severe depression, and mental sensation that can only be described as "brain fog." It left her hazy, confused, and overwhelmed. Skin rashes, bloating, and severe constipation, sharing time with burning diarrhea, also made her life miserable. "On top of all that," she laments, "I woke up one day to the pain of an exploding cyst on one of my ovaries. I'd previously been unaware of it." One thing after another, her whole system was coming unglued. Even certain smells would make her nauseous.

Early on, before things had become so completely over-whelming and out of hand, Debbie had sought the counsel of a doctor. "At first it felt like I had the flu. No fever, but very fatigued. When it lasted a couple weeks, I saw the doctor. He chalked it up to a long flu. When it was still going after two months, I saw the doctor again. Again his best guess was the flu. Frustrating!"

Eventually, Debbie heard about a doctor who specialized in figuring out what was really wrong with people when general-practice doctors or even specialists couldn't. He called his brand of care "third line" medicine.

"He took a stool sample and told me I had a ton of yeast, also known as candida, growing unchecked in my body. It was a relief to finally put a label on what my problem was." It's hard to win a war when you don't know what you're fighting. Finally, the enemy had been identified.

The antifungal medication Nystatin was prescribed, but only seemed to increase the intensity of her symptoms. Although this is quite common when first going to bat against candida—it tends to fight back—she decided to discontinue its use. Besides, at that time she wasn't completely convinced that enough safety testing had been done on what was a new drug.

"I started doing other things to tear down the yeast and, at the same time, work to build up my immune system. Liquid garlic does both. I used a product called Kyolic. I also experimented with a lot of other products, including a grapefruit extract called Paracan-myc powder, hydrochloric acid pills, and a product called SuperOxy Plus. Products containing lots of bifidus and acidophilus were also part of my program. These are good bacteria to restore what had been destroyed by the yeast in my digestive system."

Diet and exercise were also key players on the team of therapies Debbie assembled to help her win back her health. As far as diet went, she avoided a host of things, including yeast, sugar, fruit (at least at the beginning), dairy products, vinegar, mushrooms or anything that might have mold on it, anything aged, or anything refined. Meat was okay, at least according to this diet, but because of her mother's influence she was moving toward vegetarianism.

Speaking of her mother, Debbie credits this patient woman as being her "saving grace" in the midst of this war. "Mom studied up on candida and was extremely supportive. Her own health had fallen apart at one point in her life, so she knew what I was going through. I'd wake up in the middle of the night bawling, 'I can't take it any more. God doesn't love me. He's not really there.' And she'd say to me, 'I know. I understand. I've felt that way before.' I needed that kind of patience and understanding. Some people can empathize with you for a week if you've got the flu, but it's hard for them to understand when you're sick for three years. Mom was wonderful."

Boyfriend Rick, now husband Rick, was also supportive, although it didn't come easy for him at first. It was in the midst of their early dating relationship that candida first made its presence known in Debbie's system. "Our dates would be me lying on the couch and him lying on the floor, and us talking. When he asked me to marry him, we still didn't know what was wrong with me."

When it came down to diet changes and natural health-care practices to beat back this yeast, it was all new for Rick. But he was willing to learn. Love can be a tremendous motivator. " It helped him to study candida with my mother, plus he did a wealth of research on his own. In fact, he wrote a whole paper on it for one of his college classes. There was a lot of love and commitment on his part."

But back to the issue of diet and exercise, it was real important that Debbie leave out certain foods from her menu and equally important that she take in oxygen. "I was encouraged to walk outside as much as I could and to take deep breaths. Oxygen kills off yeast, plus the exercise got my circulation going so I'd eliminate more. More yeast would come out. I always noticed that I felt a lot better when I was outside."

Other elements were important to her battle plan as well. For instance, thirty minutes of sunshine a day was recommended to help stimulate the production of vitamin D. And lots of purified water was consumed to help keep her cells and organs clean. She was also encouraged to surround herself with things that would make her happy. That was difficult. In fact, in large measure the stressors she and Rick were working through as their dating relationship developed kept her body from healing itself of the candida as quickly as it might have otherwise. Stress is a notorious drain on the immune system.

Nevertheless, law and order was finally restored in Debbie's metabolic system. Balance was once more achieved. Yeast, always present in our bodies, sometimes gets out of control. Birth control pills will tip the scales toward a yeast power play. So will steroids. But for Debbie, as it has been for countless others, the genesis of her yeast problems began with taking antibiotics. "I grew up overseas where the answer to everything was antibiotics." Is the U.S. any different?

What is she doing to keep such a mutiny from ever occurring again?

"Because of what we've learned about nutrition, we're heading in the direction of a vegetarian diet. We don't buy meat or dairy for home, although sometimes we'll eat them if we go out. Even that, we're slowly trying to reduce. And of course it goes without saying that I'll be more careful about ever using antibiotics again." Today Debbie Louthan is looking good, feeling great, and running 3-5 times a week in training for a triathalon next summer.

QUOTES

"More of our populace is ill with candidiasis than anybody ever imagined. The Candida syndrome is rampant all over the world, especially in industrialized countries."

—Abram Hoffer, M.D., Ph.D.
THE YEAST SYNDROME

"A new medical condition . . . is affecting approximately $1/3$ of the total populations of all Western industrialized countries. The new disease involves a generalized yeast infection . . . commonly called Candida albicans . . . which gives rise to a loosely defined syndrome—a series of chronic disorders variably affecting the 9 different body systems: digestive, nervous, cardiovascular, lymphatic, respiratory, reproductive, urinary, endocrine, and musculoskeletal."

—John P. Trowbridge, M.D.
THE YEAST SYNDROME

"In the fall of 1979, I learned from C. Orian Truss, MD, of the relationship of Candida albicans, a common yeast, to many chronic illnesses. . . . I began treating some of my difficult patients with a special diet and the safe, antifungal medication, Nystatin. Nearly all were adults with complex health problems, including headache, fatigue, depression, irritability, digestive disorders, respiratory disorders, joint pains, skin rashes, menstrual disorders, loss of sex interest, recurrent bladder and vaginal infections and sensitivity to chemical odors and additives. Almost without exception, they improved. And some improved dramatically."

—William G. Crook, M.D.
THE YEAST CONNECTION

FURTHER READING

Back to Health: Yeast Control by Dennis W. Remington, M.D., and Barbara W. Higa, R.D. (Provo, UT: Vitality House International, Inc., 1986).

The Missing Diagnosis by C. Orian Truss, M.D. (Birmingham, AL: The Missing Diagnosis, Inc., 1982)

The Yeast Connection by William G. Crook, M.D. (Jackson, TN: Professional Books, 1986-Third Edition).

The Yeast Syndrome by John P. Trowbridge, M.D., and Morton Walker, D.P.M. (New York, NY: Bantam Books, 1986).

Who Killed Candida? by Vicki Glassburn (Brushton, NY: TEACH Service, 1991).

NOTE
1. John P. Trowbridge, M.D., *The Yeast Syndrome* (New York: Bantam Books, 1986), pages xvi-xvii.

NUTRITION AND CARDIOVASCULAR PROBLEMS

INTRODUCTION TO CARDIOVASCULAR PROBLEMS

"Forty million people in this country [the U.S.] suffer from diagnosed cardiovascular disease, and an even larger number don't yet know that they have a heart problem. Sixty million people have high blood pressure. Eighty million people have elevated cholesterol levels. Over 1.5 million Americans have heart attacks every year. And for almost one third of them, having a heart attack was their first indication that they had a heart problem—clearly not the best way to find out."[1]

It's an obvious fact of life that in the United States cardiovascular problems are the great nemesis of health. Fifty percent of Americans will die of them. Some, like the people whose stories follow, have found a way to win back their hearts and their health.

BOB NAGY

Bob Nagy's life changed forever on April 10, 1991, the day of his heart attack. He remembers saying to his wife, "I'm in big trouble. You'd better call someone." The rest is a blur of pain and fear. Nagy is one of the lucky ones. He survived his heart attack vowing to change his habits and beat America's number-one killer. Today he's in the best shape he's been in for years—eating a vegetarian diet, exercising, and eliminating stress from his life.

Nagy, of Denver, Colorado, is fifty-five years old. It's hard to believe this physically fit man once carried over 200 pounds on his 5'10" frame and had a cholesterol reading of 238. As he drizzles vinegar on his green salad, he recalls how he used to eat eight-egg omelets with a half-pound of bacon for breakfast. He also often ate a salami sandwich before bedtime. Though his blood pressure and stress levels were high, Nagy ignored warning signs of his impending heart attack.

"My dad is eighty-two and has no arterial blockage. Also, there's no history of heart disease in my family. So when I started to get some pains in my chest, I dismissed them," he recalls. "I also began having shortness of breath, which I thought was because I was getting older."

Besides his diet, Nagy believes his job increased stress and aggravated his high blood pressure. A traveling salesman, Nagy saw his company fail. Coworkers were laid off, and he knew in time he, too, would receive a pink slip. "I could see my world disintegrating," he says. "I started to worry, and as things got worse, I became impatient. Practically anything could get me upset, and I'd lose my cool."

During the night of April 10, 1991, Nagy awoke with what he thought was severe indigestion. The heart attack hit later that morning, he recalls. After a helicopter ride from his home in the foothills of the Rocky Mountains to Porter Hospital in Denver, Nagy was placed in intensive care and given pain killers. Tests revealed his left anterior descending artery was 99 percent blocked. Three days later, Nagy began having another heart attack. His physician immediately performed an angioplasty, a surgery to open blocked arteries. The procedure was successful; however, Nagy's doctor cautioned him there was a 30 percent chance his arteries would clog again.

Nagy entered the South Denver Cardiac Rehabilitation Clinic. His days were soon filled with classes in stress management, nutrition, and physical exercise. He changed his eating habits by cutting down on his portions, eliminating beef and eating only fish and skinless turkey breast. He gradually started to lose weight.

Only three months later, as his doctor predicted, Nagy needed another angioplasty. During the procedure, Nagy's doctor found another clogged blood vessel he had missed the first time. Other places in his heart were at least 50 percent blocked. Because of the degree of blockage in one artery the doctor warned that Nagy might soon require open heart surgery.

"That's when I became serious—really serious," Nagy says. Bolstering his resolve to beat this thing was a series of lectures Nagy attended. One featured Dean Ornish, M.D., whose heart-disease reversal program features no medication or surgery, with astonishing results. Another spotlighted the work of John McDougall, M.D., who recommends a low-fat vegetarian diet to treat and help prevent a variety of diseases.

"I learned things about digestion, how to read labels and how the body burns fat," Nagy says. He decided to become a vegetarian, eliminate cheese and eggs, eat more fiber, and reduce his fat intake to around 10 percent of his total calories. He hoped with dietary changes his arteries would unclog naturally and he could discontinue most of his medications.

Nagy and his wife, Cheryl, attended vegetarian and low-fat cooking classes and support groups to learn how to reduce fat in their diet. Cheryl learned to cook an entirely different way. "I can't give my wife enough credit. When we're home she eats what I eat. She's even lost weight—ten pounds," Nagy says. "We've learned to bake cakes using applesauce instead of shortening, and we now use three fat-free bread recipes."

Since his heart attack, Nagy believes his life has turned around. He exercises four times a week for two hours a session. He's lost over fifty pounds, and his cholesterol level has dropped sixty-four points to 174. Although he hasn't been retested to determine the plaque level in his arteries, the medical professionals at the rehabilitation center assure him that based on his performance on the treadmill, he's in the first stages of heart disease reversal.

Nagy says his biggest challenge has been changing his mental attitude. "I knew I had to reduce my stress level," he says.

So, he stabilized his finances and went into business for himself. He and his wife sold their mountain home and paid all their outstanding bills. They moved into a retirement community where they'll live until they retire and move back to Cheryl's family farm in South Dakota.

"I don't read newspapers or watch television except for a little PBS. I try to keep positive," Nagy says. "The most important aspect is attitude. Then there's food and exercise. I've taken control of my situation. I realize something could still happen to me, but I'll have a good feeling knowing I gave it Bob Nagy's best shot." He has found balance in his life.

To reader's who have had a heart attack, Nagy has this advice:

▲ Keep in contact with people with experiences similar to yours. They can offer support. If there's not a support group in your area, start one yourself. Find people who are interested in exercising and eating properly.

▲ Take a serious look at what you eat and make necessary changes.

▲ Keep balance in your life among diet, exercise, and especially attitude.[2]

Bob tells more of his story: "I just came from rehab this morning. I wound up talking to the fellow next to me on the treadmill. Talk about a mess. He'd had aneurysms (ballooning out) on both the outside and inside of his heart. It took five bypasses. For thirty-seven days he was in a coma. Now here he was working out in the gym, he's lost forty pounds, and he's following Dean Ornish's low-fat diet. Amazing!"

According to the vast majority of scientific studies, a low-fat diet is vital in protecting against or reversing heart disease. And eating vegetarian—removing meat and dairy products—can be an important first step. "Vegetarian cooking in itself, however, can still involve lots of fat," Bob points out. "The real trick is to learn how to prepare vegetarian meals that truly are low-fat or no-fat."

So how does one do that? How would a person who is interested in changing to a healthier diet go about learning how? Bob and Cheryl have developed their new lifestyle and eating habits by reading books and taking advantage of local seminars and support groups. "Our diet just evolved as we took in everything available and learned what we could. We've discovered that no one program is the 100 percent right approach for everyone. We've simply opened ourselves up like sponges, absorbing as much of the information out there from as many sources as we possibly could. Then we've tried things and stuck with what works for us."

A low-fat, totally vegetarian diet is what is working for Bob these days. He feels very good about the changes he's made, but it hasn't been easy.

"It's a real challenge, especially when you're in the kind of business that I'm in. I'm always taking clients out to lunch. They order a big steak. I order a salad and put a little lemon juice on it instead of dressing. First they look at me like I'm a leper. Then, when they find out why I'm eating this way, I become the center of conversation. Finally, they all start feeling guilty. Actually, these changes in my eating habits have involved a real maturing process for me. I know what's right for me, and I try to do it regardless of what others think."

Eating the way Bob now eats can, indeed, be a challenge to one's creativity and discipline. It would be much easier for him to fall back into past habits. The thing is, he's tasted what it's like to be healthy. It tastes good.

"The success of my diet changes," he enthuses, "have been dynamite! There are, of course, no guarantees, but I certainly feel a whole lot better about myself. One of the neatest things is to be off most of the medications. I feel like I'm driving the car again, not just a passenger in a bus waiting for things to happen. For me, it's a lot like selling. Success breeds success. The first sale is always the hardest, but then you think 'Hey, I can do this.' Things start to snowball. You build a big success on top of a lot of little successes. One step at a time."

JUDITH MARTIN

Judith Martin was living out her dream. From the age of nine on, her passion had been performance. She loved the theater, the stage, the audience. That world had become her world.

"The future seemed bright and glittering when I was twenty-two," she recalls. "Success was easy, obstacles were few. Propelled by the invincibility of youth, I was sure my destiny rested in my own hands. My daughter, Kathryn, had just been born. Getting married and having a child was a short detour from my main objective: a career on stage."

Six weeks after Kathryn's birth, Judith was back performing with a local theatrical company. One night she stood at center stage and began to sing.

"My lungs suddenly felt constricted; breathing became difficult. Panic surged through my body as I struggled to finish the performance. A doctor examined me the following day and said my symptoms indicated a classic case of 'nervous young mother,' nothing more."

What he failed to identify was the deadly virus that was in the process of attacking the outer layer of tissue around Judith's heart. Hospitalized several weeks later, her heart had swelled out to her ribs. Forty-two pounds of excess water had collected in her tissues. Test results revealed that 76 percent of her heart had sustained damaged. She was given no hope to live.

Thirty years later, Judith is still in the land of the living. Although her heart remains in critical condition, she continues to squeeze maximum life out of minimum days.

"My doctors keep telling me they've never seen anyone live as long as I have with a condition like mine," she says with the air of a humble, yet conquering warrior. "Day to day they don't expect me to live. My heart doesn't pump enough blood to support life, but God just keeps me going." Indeed, God seems to play a central role in Judith's battle plan to win back her health. But this wasn't always the case.

From age twenty-two to thirty-five, Judith found herself in a constant trudge in and out of hospital beds and wheelchairs. Those were dark and desperate years for her. Although she was surrounded by loved ones who cared, she found life slipping through her hands. Where once there had been a woman with ambition and passion— a budding performer playing to theaters filled with adoring fans—

now there was a shell of a person haunted by a sense of emptiness and fear—fear of being out of control over her life and out of touch with its purpose.

By the time she turned thirty-five, Judith knew that something inside her needed to change, and not just her heart. It had to do with her soul. She reached out to touch someone, someone whom she hoped would touch her back. It was the first time in her life when she was willing to open herself up to God.

What followed was not lightning bolts and fire alarms. The Red Sea didn't part again, nor was health immediately restored to her. What did happen was that her mind was invaded by a calm assurance that her body was not hers alone, that it belonged also to Another.

"I began to ask God what to do about my health. I loved to eat fried foods, even after my heart had gotten so bad and I was confined to a wheelchair. I began to realize that I had allowed my belly to rule my life, to be my god. It took me two years to admit that to myself."

By degrees, a little at a time over the next ten years, Judith began to develop better eating habits. She wanted to put the kinds of foods into her body that would help her heart, not hurt it. "I started eating more fresh fruits and vegetables," she says, "even though I was still hanging on to some of the things I knew I shouldn't—like meat, dairy, and processed foods."

Even so, things were getting better. Her health was gradually improving. Putting aside her wheelchair and resuming the normal activities of a busy wife and mother, she even went to work in the bicycle shop with husband, Butch, and fifteen-year-old Kathryn. It wasn't unusual to find Judith there six days a week, eleven hours a day. Even though her heart was still dramatically enlarged and severely damaged, her energy and stamina were remarkable.

Then came another turning point. Although her eating habits had improved over that ten-year period, they were not yet what they could have been. Intestinal disturbances plagued her. A change in the family business had also been undertaken. They were now running a computerized income tax service. Unbeknownst to all, a copying machine in the new office was giving off toxic fumes that were significantly affecting Judith. Her health began to fail badly once more.

Again she turned to God for help, and two days later she discovered the book *Fit for Life* by Harvey and Marilyn Diamond. It taught her much about a health-promoting diet, including the importance of combining foods correctly.

The Diamonds teach that different foods require different digestive fluids in order to be effectively broken down and assimilated by the body. For instance, proteins should not be consumed with starches. A steak, which requires an acidic digestive juice, should not be consumed with a potato, which requires an alkaline juice. If eaten together the two juices neutralize each other. The body is then forced to invest a huge amount of energy to try to get this mixture broken down and out of the stomach. After several hours, and without ever fully digesting its contents, the stomach hands off to the intestines—"Here, you take it." The result is a putrefied, fermenting mass of stuff making its way through one's intestines, causing gas, flatulence, heartburn, acid indigestion, malabsorption, and a call for relief, R-O-L-A-I-D-S.

Another important food-combining principle put forth in *Fit for Life* involves eating fruit twenty minutes before anything else, or all by itself as a meal or snack. Fruit digests so rapidly that if eaten in conjunction with anything else, it will sit atop the other food and ferment.

The Diamonds, as well as most nutritionally aware professionals, caution people about the hazards of consuming animal products—meat and dairy. These are high in fat, low in fiber, hard for the body to digest, and in this day and age, heavily contaminated by concentrated levels of pollutants and production chemicals. And then there's the problem of cholesterol in all animal products—not something a hurting heart needs to deal with.

At the same time when Judith was learning about food combining and the benefits of a vegetarian diet, she happened to attend a seminar put on by Dr. Mary Ruth Swope, author of *Green Leaves of Barley*. Here she heard for the first time about the amazing benefits of chlorophyll—that it helps to build and clean the blood, bolster the immune system, and enhance absorption and utilization of nutrients, among other things.

"Dr. Swope's words were just what I needed to hear. I got to talk with her personally about my situation, and she suggested that I do a nine-month internal cleanse. I began to eat nothing but fresh fruit and vegetables, water, juice, and a product rich in chlorophyll called Barley Green. I also took an enzyme called CoQ10, which helps to strengthen the heart. I ate nothing canned, frozen, or otherwise processed—and very little cooked. I got a steamer. Anything I wanted warm, I lightly steamed.

"Two months into this regime I woke up one morning with a large oval shaped blister next to my navel. The next day I was broken out all over my stomach, back, head, and face. At fifty-one years of age, I was experiencing the chicken pox. My mother had told me that when I was five I'd been exposed to them but, unlike all the other kids, I never developed the illness. Obviously the virus had been in my system all this time, but my liver had been unable to flush it from my body. Now, with the help of a new diet, new principles of eating, and Barley Green, my body was beginning to clean itself out."

Today Judith is feeling great. "I've never felt like this before in my entire life!" she says with enthusiasm. "I feel just marvelous! I really believe that my body is in a rebuilding stage. The first stage was the flushing and tissue cleansing. Now I'm rebuilding and excited about how God is leading me step by step back to better health. I don't know what will happen with my heart. It remains enlarged and in critical condition, but I do walk, go up and down stairs every day, and maintain an active lifestyle. I just don't stop to think about it."

Judith's dream of a life on stage was short lived. Today, however, she lives out another. "I love talking to people about their health, both physical and spiritual. I have many opportunities to be of help and encouragement."

Judith Martin does have a big heart—a big heart to help people around her who are suffering. A heart to help people get healthy, both physically and spiritually. In that light she's written a book of her own entitled *Peace in the Face of Death*. She knows the territory.

DALE WILLARD

Over the first sixty-three years of his life, Dale Willard's health history read like a medical textbook. Pneumonia, digestion problems, sinus infections and headaches, lengthy periods of fatigue and depression, prostatitis (prostate problems), bleeding ulcer, kidney stones, allergies, high blood pressure, constipation and diarrhea, gall bladder problems, acid reflux problems, hernia, insomnia, hemorrhoids, and osteoarthritis. Significant health concerns seemed to dog him at every turn. Physically he was falling apart at the seams. The grayish coloring in his skin gave away the secret that all was not well. Emotionally, he was hanging on by a thread.

One day his wife happened to bring home a book Anne and I wrote called *A Cancer Battle Plan.* "Twenty-four hours later, I'd read that thing from cover to cover, including the cover! Although I didn't have cancer, reading the book convinced me that proper nutrition would be a great help in any abnormal physical condition." Goodness knows, he had plenty to choose from. He was so frustrated with his health situation that he was ready to try almost anything.

For the first time in his life, Dale sought the help of a professional nutritionist. A lengthy medical history was taken, the essential first step in any health-care program that seeks to address and remedy the cause of an ailment, not just treat the symptoms. Several potential sources of his health problems were identified. A program of supplements was tailor made to help address these, and a meat-and-dairy–free diet of organic fruits, vegetables, and grains was initiated.

"I had been off animal products about a month," Dale recalls, "when I rolled out of bed one morning and realized that my joints didn't hurt and my legs weren't stiff. For years it had been the exact opposite."

Animal products, by the way, are high in protein. High protein diets rob the body of calcium, which can lead to the onset of arthritic symptoms and osteoporosis (bone loss). (See *Healthy Habits*, chapter 6.)

In the process of refining his diet, Dale also discovered that there were certain vegetables that he needed to avoid, at least for the foreseeable future. Cabbage, broccoli, Brussels sprouts, and cauliflower all seemed to bring with them flare-ups in his arthritic symptoms. "Those vegetables had a negative effect on my thyroid," explains Dale. "And according to my nutritionist, there is a direct connection between thyroid complications and arthritis."

Thank goodness for those professionals who are trained to help us make sense out of the complexity of our individually unique biochemistry. Adopting a vegetarian diet helped Dale gain control of his arthritis, but even this needed fine tuning to match the special needs of his particular metabolic system.

In addition to changing his eating habits, Dale also set about the process of detoxifying his body, sort of like spring cleaning. Years of eating the standard American diet and being exposed to the chemicals and other pollutants in the environment had taken their toll. The effectiveness of his immune system had no doubt been compromised by the buildup of toxins in his cells.

Where to start? Clean the colon. "I went to a colonic therapist for a colon irrigation. During the procedure, she detected yeast (otherwise known as candida) in what was coming out of me."

Yeast overgrowth in a person's system can be very destructive (refer to the chapter on candida). One of the most dangerous things it can do is to keep the intestinal tract from absorbing nutrients from food. Regardless of the quality of cuisine consumed, the body is slowly starved of what it needs to function at peak performance. Not only did Dale's nutritionist put him on some things to help combat the yeast, but she also did a hair analysis to check on specific nutrient balances in his system. Sure enough, the test showed that he was deficient in ten out of fourteen essential minerals.

"I gradually worked up to the maximum dosage of nine capsules a day of the anti-yeast supplement, and at the same time began taking four capsules a day of the multi-mineral supplement," Dale recalls. "After the second day of the mineral supplement, I had a better sense of well-being than I'd had for years."

At that point, things were looking up. Progress had been made on several fronts. Diet changes were helping to deal with the pain and frustrations associated with arthritis. An effective war was also being waged against the yeast invaders in his intestinal tract. Nutrient supplies were beginning to make their way through enemy resistance to reinforce his efforts to win back his health.

"I felt stronger and had a better outlook on life. My digestion was better than it *ever* had been. My old problems of constipation and diarrhea were practically nonexistent. I had lost some weight, primarily in my waist. And I had successfully reduced the amount of medication I was taking for allergies, essentially discontinuing the steroid nasal spray. I couldn't help but believe that this whole series of events was an answer to our prayers for guidance in the area of improving our health."

But still, Dale had a long way to go. He had no sense of having "arrived." Those occasional days of fatigue and depression for no apparent reason reminded him that the battle for his health had not yet turned completely in his favor. There were more enemies to be faced and conquered.

Perhaps the most sinister of these tipped its hand one day while Dale was out working in his yard. "I was planting flowers in our garden when I first noticed it. Chest pains."

Anybody who knows anything about health, knows that chest pains are not something to be taken lightly. *Angina*, a fancy word for them, can be a sign of a heart in distress—a heart that's not functioning properly because of restricted blood supply.

The first medical doctor Dale saw about his chest pains failed to uncover any cause. "He did an EKG and looked at blood work," Dale recalls. "And from that he decided I was healthy. Nothing to worry about. The problem was, the chest pains kept getting worse. It got to the point where I couldn't walk half a block vigorously without fatigue and nausea."

That certainly didn't sound like someone who had nothing to worry about. What now? Perhaps something could be done to remedy the pains nutritionally. No luck. The pains continued. But through the network he had established with nutrition experts, Dale was eventually linked up with an M.D. who was not only able to identify his problem, but also respected his desire to deal with it as non-invasively as possible.

"He put me on a treadmill test, something the first guy didn't, and within two minutes detected irregularities. We went ahead with an angiogram and discovered that one of the arteries that supplies blood to my heart was completely clogged. There was no indication of heart damage, however. And on that basis, he highly recommended that I bypass bypass surgery and go with chelation therapy and diet, instead."

Chelation therapy involves an intravenous drip of a solution called EDTA—a synthetic amino acid—accompanied with nutrients such as magnesium, vitamin B-complex, and vitamin C. It's used to help remove heavy metal poisoning from blood, but has also been shown in hundreds of published medical studies to be effective at dissolving and flushing away plaque buildup in arteries, a condition known as atherosclerosis. A single treatment takes between three to four hours. A series of such treatments is required for full effect. Although the FDA approves of chelation therapy for heavy metal poisoning, it has been slow to put its full stamp of approval on the same for circulatory problems. Doctors who use chelation therapy in this way run the potential risk of FDA reprisal. With the coverage chelation is getting in the medical media these days, however, it may not be long before consumers push bypass surgery off to one side and demand that chelation therapy become "king of the hill."

Dale Willard is one of those willing to do some pushing. "The doctor tells me that there's about an 85 percent chance that chelation will clear out my clogged artery. I'm already seeing great improvement. After eleven treatments, my circulation has improved dramatically. My hands and feet, in the past always cold, are warm. The color in my face is better than it's been for years. I can now exercise without chest pains. And even my vision has been improving. I'm just thanking God that the first doctor I saw didn't put me on the treadmill. Had he done so and found my problem, he'd have probably stuck me in the hospital for bypass surgery on the spot."

And so what's to be said about diet and nutrition in the midst of all this about chelation therapy?

"My doctor told me that I was one of the 10 percent lucky ones not to have suffered a massive heart attack with an artery closed up like mine. It got that way because I used to eat a lot of fat in my diet. I firmly believe that my situation wasn't as bad as it could have been because of the vegetarian diet I had recently adopted. In fact, my doctor was thrilled to death when he heard about our dietary changes. In addition, he suggested a more sophisticated water filtering system, more than just the simple carbon block filter we'd been using. Carbon block filters alone don't remove fluoride. He sees a strong connection between fluoride and heart disease, along with other degenerative problems. It's obviously not the only thing, but an important contributor."

Dale Willard, a man out to help his heart. He's come a long way, and perhaps has a ways still to go, but at least he knows he's on the right track.

QUOTES

William Castelli, M.D., of the well-known Framingham Heart Study was asked to identify the optimal diet for a healthy heart. His reply, "Vegetarians have the best."

"In 1989, an estimated 944,688 Americans died because of cardiovascular disease (CVD). That's one death every 32 seconds. And death is only part of the tragedy. About 1.5 million people suffer and/or die from heart attacks each year. Nearly 500,000 more have CVD-related strokes. And then there are the countless hours of misery spent in surgery, in painful recovery, in disability, in a family's grief, and in worry about how to pay the bills. CVD's financial cost to our economy and our health system in 1992 alone was a staggering $108.9 billion. . . . We can stop this epidemic in its tracks. . . . Researchers are teaching us that all we have to do is to change our lifestyles and nutrition."
—Terry T. Shintani, M.D.
52 WAYS TO PREVENT HEART DISEASE

"A diet high in saturated fat and cholesterol provides the building blocks for coronary atherosclerosis. The role of diet in heart disease has been studied for years. What's new is that we now know diet affects the heart very quickly, not just over a period of years. Even a single meal high in fat and cholesterol may cause the body to release a hormone, thromboxane, which causes the

arteries to constrict and the blood to clot faster. . . . The good news is that improvements also can occur very quickly. . . . We can make different lifestyle choices to begin healing ourselves. In our research, we found that blood flow to the heart could begin to improve in just a few weeks. Our diet allowed participants' arteries to dilate and blood to flow more freely because the fat and cholesterol content was so low."

—Dean Ornish, M.D.
DR. DEAN ORNISH'S PROGRAM FOR REVERSING HEART DISEASE

"Chelation has been used safely over 6 million times in over 400,000 patients in the US alone. Its success rate in improving blood flow in patients with clogged arteries is close to 82%."

—Elmer Cranton, M.D.
BYPASSING BYPASS

FURTHER READING

Bypassing Bypass by Elmer Cranton, M.D., and Arline Brecher (Trout Dale, VA: Medex Publishers, Inc., 1990).

The Chelation Way by Dr. Morton Walker (Garden City Park, NY: Avery Publishing Group, 1990).

Dr. Dean Ornish's Program for Reversing Heart Disease by Dean Ornish, M.D. (New York: Ballantine Books, 1990).

Eradicating Heart Disease by Matthias Rath, M.D. (San Francisco, CA: Health Now, 1993).

NOTES
1. Dean Ornish, M.D., *Dr. Dean Ornish's Program for Reversing Heart Disease* (New York, NY: Ballantine Books, 1990), page 11.
2. *Acknowledgment:* The previous section of Bob Nagy's story appeared in *Delicious!* (a magazine dedicated to health and natural living), February 1994. It was written by Gloria Bucco. Permission for its use was granted by *Delicious*, Gloria Bucco, and by Bob Nagy. The section that follows is an interview I conducted with Bob Nagy.

NUTRITION AND DIABETES

INTRODUCTION TO DIABETES

The disease commonly referred to as diabetes affects close to 5% of the US population, and about 10% of those over 60. It is estimated that there are about 12 million diabetics in the country, both diagnosed and undiagnosed.

Medical dictionaries actually list many forms of diabetes, but when we talk about diabetes in common terms we use the term to mean the disease *diabetes mellitus*, sometimes called "sugar diabetes." "Diabetes" is a combined term that comes from the Greek words for "to go through"—and indeed, frequent urination is a major symptom of this disease. "Mellitus" comes from the Greek word for honey.

Basically, diabetes mellitus is a disorder of the body's means of utilizing sugar, or glucose—the body's basic fuel. Before the food we eat can be used as fuel by our muscles and other body tissues, it must first be converted into glucose. Then, the glucose must enter the individual cells where it is metabolized, or "burned" to provide energy for the cell's functions. The hormone insulin, which is manufactured by the islet cells of the pancreas, is necessary for glucose utilization to occur.[1]

There are two types of diabetes mellitus, type 1 (juvenile-onset, insulin dependent) and type 2 (adult-onset, non-insulin dependent).

DEBBIE CORNELL

"I knew that complications were possible," admits Debbie Cornell, "but I just never figured they'd happen to me."

At the tender age of eleven, Debbie learned she had diabetes. Her weight had steadily dropped to a mere seventy pounds, and her energy level had all but bottomed out. A stay in the local hospital revealed the news. She would need daily insulin shots for the rest of her life.

A routine was quickly established, and for years she seemed to be doing fine. In fact, she reveled in the feeling of being on top of her condition and in control of the disease. She gave little thought to what other things she could be doing to bolster her health.

"I'd been told about what sort of things could happen down the line, but I was playing Queen of Denial. Not me. Those kinds of things weren't going to happen to me!"

Somewhere about fifteen years into her battle, though, things started to get dicey. "I developed a condition called retinopathy—buildup of blood vessels in the back of the eye. These can pop and cause blindness. I guess I was on my way that direction. Laser surgery, however, helped stave off that potential."

A few years down the road, more breakdowns in her system began to occur.

"I started to have kidney problems, a common complication for diabetics. One month I put on thirty pounds of water weight. Still, the denial ran deep. I'd look in the mirror and tell myself that it wasn't really that much weight. I always gained weight with my periods. Intellectually I knew I was in real trouble and headed for dialysis, but psychologically, I just refused to accept the reality of my condition. I was one of those people who said, 'No machine is going to keep me alive.'"

Debbie did her best to keep on her feet that month, but at times it took all the energy she could muster just to get out of bed and go to the bathroom. Going to work was next to impossible. Ironically, she worked at the local hospital as a neuropsychological technician, testing head injuries—the same hospital where she finally checked herself in to begin dialysis.

"I ultimately had to face up to the truth about my condition."

To be in a position to need dialysis is not fun. As Debbie explains it, "There is a certain component, creatinine, that's analyzed in blood chemistry that tells how a person's kidneys are doing. Normal people will be at .5 to 1.5. Without dialysis I was at sixteen—real, real sick. With dialysis I was at nine—just real sick. Dialysis can keep you alive indefinitely, but at the same time definitely sick. It helps to clean your blood, but not nearly as well as healthy kidneys. One thing it doesn't do is remove potassium. Therefore, eating a bunch of bananas or potatoes could have killed me. My heart would've gone into arrythmia. I had to avoid most fruit and vegetables."

In the midst of her health woes, Debbie's sister, Charlene, presented her with a gift—the kind of gift that fellow dialysis patients are just dying to receive. It was a kidney. A perfectly matched kidney. Twenty years into her war, she was being given new ammo.

This is where the story turns toward nutrition.

"I'd always read books on nutrition, but had really never had much interest in practicing any of what I learned. One complication I was experiencing from the kidney failure was that I was developing cataracts, clouding of the lens in the eye. Professionals don't know why that happens, but that it does is very, very frustrating. It's like trying to see through a coating of Vaseline. Emotionally, it was much harder for me to deal with this than with the kidney situation. Again I couldn't read. In fact, I could barely see at all. And getting the new kidney was not going to help. The ophthalmologist told me that the only way to deal with cataracts was more surgery. Without it, my eyes wouldn't get any better, but probably worse.

"Well, in the books I'd been reading, I came across stories of people who had gotten rid of cataracts through nutritional therapies.

I decided to try it. I got a book called *Prescription for Nutritional Healing* by James F. Balch, M.D., and his wife, Phyllis A. Balch, a nutritionist, and followed closely the program they outlined for self treatment of cataracts."

And did it work?

"I can see now! My vision isn't what it used to be, but I can drive and read again. I had to retake my driving test, and I passed just fine. The doctor had said that my eyes would not get better without surgery, but they did. Among other things, I took mega-doses of vitamins A, B-complex, and C, together with calcium, magnesium, and zinc. It's all spelled out in that book, and it helped me improve my vision.

"Nutrition has also helped me lower my cholesterol and triglyc-erides from 500 and 400 respectively, to 160 and 70. Even with kidney transplants, a lot of people still have cholesterol levels in the 300's."

Although she's had to be on immunosuppressant drugs to keep her immune system from rejecting the new kidney, Debbie has not been sick one day since the transplant—over four years ago.

"Not even a cold. Nothing! Along with the vitamin C, I take Kyolic garlic. It's an excellent antiviral, antifungal, antibacterial agent. Together with vitamin C, they're a great one-two punch. Bioflavinoids to strengthen blood vessels, and several different kinds of herbs are also part of my program. I take these and the rest of my supplements three times a day without fail. I never miss."

Debbie's been through some pretty tough times in her battle with diabetes. Her hope is to be of service to others who are in the same war, especially kids. "It's hard enough to go through all this at thirty," she says, "I can't imagine going through it as a child." She's planning to go back to school for a Ph.D. in child psychology.

And what would she tell kids and their parents about nutrition?

"I just talked to a man today whose child, a six-year-old, had recently been diagnosed with diabetes. I didn't get the chance, but I wanted to tell him to get this kid on a program of diet and sup-plements. If he does, I strongly believe there's a good chance of avoiding all the complications associated with diabetes. It just makes sense, looking at it biochemically. But no one's telling him that. No one told me that. I really wish I had done this nutritional stuff while I was a teenager. But at that stage, I just figured the shots were enough. Obviously, they weren't." In the end Debbie has this to say about her health: "I'm alive because I've had a transplant; I'm healthy because of what I do nutritionally. There are a lot of people who have had transplants who aren't healthy."

Author's Note
Debbie wanted me to add that if a diabetic takes a lot of vitamin C, it can affect blood glucose reading. It shows up too high. Also, those with transplants who take large doses of vitamin C increase potential of organ rejection because of their improved immune system.

DEBBIE LOUDENBACK
Handfuls of jelly beans. Snickers bars. Orange juice with tons of sugar in it. That used to be what it took for Debbie Loudenback to raise the blood sugar levels in her body.

"Now I can raise them with just an ordinary apple," she says with an obvious sense of accomplishment. "That doesn't happen for the average diabetic. They usually need much, much more in the way of sugary foods, like I used to. What I've learned about nutrition has really helped me gain better control over my diabetes and my body."

Debbie was seven when it was discovered that she had the disease. It was around Easter time. A virus had been at work on her body, so had sugar from a load of Easter candy. The combination of the two seemed to do a number on her pancreas, causing it to fall into disrepair.

The daughter of missionaries, Debbie was carted off to Europe just eighteen months after her diagnosis, as her parents set out for this new ministry location. It was, of course, a bit unnerving for them as they faced making a home for their family in a new country and new culture, not knowing how Debbie would respond or the quality of specialized help they'd be able to find for her.

"But over there," she recalls, "they don't let you go from the hospital until everything is perfect. I would go in for three to six weeks at a time just to change my insulin."

High school and college years were passable health-wise. There were yearly bouts with bronchitis, accompanied often by ear and sinus problems. Antibiotics were always part of the mix. But as far as the diabetes was concerned, it seemed to be under control. Debbie was careful to watch the sort of foods she ate and involved herself in sporting activities that would help keep her body in shape. "During that period of my life, I really focused on my health. I knew it was important that I took care of myself."

Unfortunately, that attitude began to wane as she reached her twenties. After college, Debbie went into the working world, and she put aside her health disciplines in favor of satisfying her sweet tooth. "I got into eating chocolate and cheese cake. Every chance I could I'd eat something sweet. I'd been so careful all those years, I just wanted to know what it was like to be free to eat whatever I wanted. I honestly didn't think it was having any impact on my diabetes. I found out later that it was."

"Later" came all too soon. At twenty-four she started to experience mysterious bouts with nausea. At twenty-six, she and husband, Brad, celebrated the birth of their son Jordan. That was the last celebrating she would do for a long, long time. For the next two years, what felt like "morning sickness" haunted her every single day. Dizziness, nausea, and fatigue were her constant companions. Brad would come home from work at five o'clock in the evening. Debbie would hand him Jordan, then head to bed for the night.

Doctors were consulted. Tests were performed. Everything from AIDS and brain tumors to hearing loss was checked for. The blood work, according to the doctors, appeared normal. Meanwhile, Debbie got sicker and weaker.

"I never thought about killing myself," she recalls, "but I do remember lots of days lying on the floor in pain, yelling at God. I was a mess!"

Just how big a mess she really was didn't become clear until she finally went to consult with a woman who was both a naturopathic doctor and a nutritionist. Now *here* was a professional who knew how to read blood. In fact, she had taught doctors how to do it.

"She took one look at my blood work and said, 'And you're still standing?!' My liver was very congested, and my adrenal glands were all but shot. In fact, she told me she'd had a friend with my same level of liver and adrenal gland functioning who had, as a result, gone into a coma." Now that bit of information would tend to get your attention!

At her urging, Debbie immediately launched herself on an aggressive program to clean out and detoxify her liver. For ten days she followed a strict dietary regime: freshly made apple juice five times a day, raw grated veggies for lunch, raw grated apples throughout the day, and a protein shake each day to help keep insulin levels stable and sugar under control. She also did an enema each day, using distilled water, acidophilus, and lemon to clean and detoxify her colon.

"At the end of this cleaning-out period, I continued with a strictly vegetarian diet—no meat, no dairy. Without the dairy in my diet, the problems I'd always had with mucus went away." So did her sinus problems and frequent bouts with bronchitis and ear infections. So bad had her sinuses gotten during her two-year tailspin that she'd had surgery. It hadn't helped. Getting off dairy products, however, did the trick.

Debbie's naturopathic doctor also employed muscle testing, a procedure for identifying allergic responses to foods and other products the body comes into contact with. "When she first tested me, I was completely overwhelmed," Debbie admits. "It seemed like I was allergic to everything, even the fresh bread I was making at home. Now I learned I couldn't have wheat, chicken, spinach, tomatoes—a whole bunch of different things. My body was just so toxic. I was even allergic to some of the things I wore, my detergents, my shampoos, conditioners, soap—all that stuff. No wonder I had been getting out of the shower too sick to even dry my hair. My liver had become congested because of the steady flow of insulin and my poor diet. All the antibiotics probably played a part, too. It was just too much for my liver to handle."

Today, however, Debbie's doing great. As she cleaned out her body and changed her diet, not only did many of her allergies vanish and respiratory problems clear up, but she regained control over her run away needs for sugar and insulin. "It's been nineteen months, and I feel absolutely incredible! I have energy, and that's new for me. The amount of insulin I need has been cut in half. When I was pregnant I was taking 150 units a day. When I started to clean up my body I was needing fifty. Now I'm down to just twenty-three. And as I said, if I need a sugar boost, an apple will do it. No more jelly beans and Snickers bars."

Debbie knows that because her pancreas doesn't function, she will always need to use insulin. And she knows that insulin is hard on her liver. "That's why it's important for me to keep it clean," she says with determination in her voice. Her plan is to do a liver flush every couple of months. The chiropractor/nutritionist she has added to her health-support team alongside her naturopathic doctor has outlined a program of apple juice, coffee enemas, a mixture of olive oil and grapefruit juice, and Epsom salts. He has also helped her expand her vegetarian diet by introducing her to a variety of new foods.

"Doctors often tell diabetics that you need your protein—meat and dairy, in other words. I have found that I can get enough protein from fruits and vegetables. My doctor back in Indianapolis would've shot me if I told him I was going vegetarian. I told my endocrinologist here what I was doing, and she said to keep doing what I was doing. I was expecting her to say, 'You need your protein.' So many professionals don't realize that vegetables and fruit have protein in them."

What would she tell others, diabetic or not, who might ask her about health issues?

"Eat natural. Avoid the processed foods. Try eliminating animal products. The more you eat like this, the more control you'll have over your health."

QUOTES

"In the United States, inappropriate diet is probably the major factor associated with insulin insensitivity and thus the major cause of diabetes."

—Julian Whitaker, M.D.
REVERSING DIABETES

"Most type 2 (or adult-onset) diabetics are overweight. Losing weight makes the body cells more responsive to the insulin that the pancreas is producing, and this change alone will 'cure' many diabetics. Regular exercise will promote weight loss, and has the further advantage of making the body's natural insulin more potent by increasing the sensitivity of the body cells. However, the most effective approach to improving diabetes is a sensible change in the body's intake of its basic sources of energy.

"Instead of the diet high in fats, proteins, and refined foods . . . switch to a low-fat diet offering much more carbohydrates and fiber. The proportions for this ideal diet are 80-90% carbohydrates, 5-12% proteins, 5-10% fats, with no cholesterol at all, and a high content of fiber. This kind of diet will reduce the blood sugar levels of most diabetics (both types). . . . Please note that this is the same sensible diet that cuts down on the amounts of those harmful components that contribute to the development of complications in diabetes, such as atherosclerosis, heart attacks, kidney failure, and blindness."

—John A. McDougall, M.D.
MCDOUGALL'S MEDICINE

"Physicians who practice alternative approaches to treating diabetes for the most part employ a program combining exercise and diet modification aimed at both better nutrition and weight loss (where this is indicated). This sort of program has been shown to have considerable success in lowering and stabilizing blood sugar levels in a very short period of time. It also reduces and frequently eliminates the various symptoms of diabetes. By displacing or cutting down the need for insulin. . . . It can help diabetic patients avoid many long-range side effects and debilitating complications."

—Gary Null
HEALING YOUR BODY NATURALLY

FURTHER READING

Healing Your Body Naturally by Gary Null (New York: Four Walls Eight Windows, 1992), see chapter 8, "Diabetes."

McDougall's Medicine by John A. McDougall, M.D. (Piscataway, NJ: New Century Publishers, 1985), see chapter 7, "Diabetes."

Reversing Diabetes by Julian M. Whitaker, M.D. (New York: Warner Books, 1987).

NOTE
1. Julian M. Whitaker, M.D., *Reversing Diabetes* (New York: Warner Books, 1987), page 3.

9

NUTRITION AND ENVIRONMENTAL ILLNESS

INTRODUCTION TO ENVIRONMENTAL ILLNESS

Today a whole new type of illness plagues modern society, promising to do even greater damage in the years ahead. The title commonly given this category of sickness is environmental illness (EI). Because the primary cause has been found to be chemical pollutants in the air one breathes and the water one drinks, the illness is sometimes also referred to as multiple chemical sensitivities (MCS).

EI is actually a form of allergy—an allergy to this century and beyond. For modern-day life finds us surrounded by manufactured products that are "outgasing" chemical fumes into our air or releasing their toxic load into our water supply. This chemical influence is nearly impossible to escape. And for those whose bodies are particularly sensitive to these conditions, life can become a living hell.

Air and water are the two most important nutrients for human health. What follows are stories of EI warriors who have found, or are in the process of finding, ways and means of obtaining the quality of air and water they need. They chart a course that thousands more like them are following. As long as pollution continues to take its toll on our world, there will be many more.

NANCY JOHNSTON
The doctor looked her in the eye and said, "Nancy, what you need if you want to get well is just two words, *clean air!*"

Hmmmm. Clean air. Not easy to come by in some parts, but vitally important for good health. Air is the most important nutrient for human life; the cleaner the better. You can get along without food for weeks and without water for days. But six minutes without air and you're a corpse. Earth is home to 6,000 billion tons of the stuff, but not all of it is fit to breathe. (See chapter 18 in *Healthy Habits*, "Breathe Clean Air.") If the air a person lives in, day in and day out, is filled with pollutants, as Nancy's had been, every cell becomes polluted. Toxic. Extreme sensitivities begin to show up to the chemicals in things like cleaning products, medications, fabrics, carpeting, gasoline fumes, detergents, perfumes, paints, adhesives, building products, and even foods. It's as if the body is saying, "Hey, I've had more than I can stand, I can stand no more!" Ultimately, the person can become sensitive—*environmentally ill* is the term used—to just about everything. Allergic to this century, as some have put it.

We've all seen the stories on "60 Minutes" and other TV shows about such people holed away like monks in the deserts of Arizona or some other barely livable place—out there away from everything but sun and sand. Perhaps you thought that those people were paranoid neurotics or weirdos looking for attention. I'm here to tell you otherwise. The EI (environmental illness) sufferers I've met and interviewed are very normal people whose only crime is a body that has accumulated a collective overdose of toxicity from their environment. There are thousands of such people.

The day that I called to interview Nancy, she'd just recovered from wounds at the hands of an unkind and arrogant dentist who didn't believe her story about chemical sensitivities.

"I'd interviewed three dentists and settled on him," she says with a great deal of disappointment evident in her voice. "I told him what sort of painkiller I could tolerate and what I couldn't. He agreed to use the stuff my system could stand, but then used something else." As a result, soon after she'd arrived home her face broke out "like someone had scalded me with fire." Her blood pressure plummeted—24/80. She was forced to take emergency measures to reclaim herself from death's doorstep.

After being sick in bed for several weeks, she finally regained enough of herself to confront the guy. "Oh," he said, "I think it was something else in your apartment building that made you sick. Maybe the carpet." But she knew the truth. Treat her like just one more silly woman if you will, but the truth is still the truth. He'd agreed to use what she could handle, then violated that promise and his patient.

This sort of uncaring treatment is not new to Nancy, nor to the thousands like her around the U.S. Environmental illness and related chemical sensitivities are perhaps the least understood of all maladies that now plague our society. Those of us whose immune systems are still strong enough to fight off the toxic impact of all the pollutants and toxins we're exposed to each day have a hard time sympathizing with those who can't. The medical world has been slow to accept the diagnosis of environmental illness; the general public even slower. Perhaps part of it has to do with the fact that those who are most susceptible to EI are women. And we all know how women are when it comes to health complaints, right? Wrong!

EI, environmental illness, is a reality. There are real reasons, scientific reasons, why sane people are getting sick from their environment. It's not just an imagined problem in the minds of a few paranoid women. If EI and its associated condition of chronic fatigue syndrome (CFS) is already a part of your life, perhaps these stories will give you some measure of help and hope.

It's possible some people still have never heard of chronic fatigue syndrome. Here's a description from world-renown author, lecturer, and medical practitioner William G. Crook, M.D.:

What is Chronic Fatigue Syndrome?
People with devastating fatigue, muscle aching, memory loss, confused thinking, digestive problems, food allergies, chemical sensitivities, and other symptoms are suffering

from a true disease (CFS). Moreover, these symptoms may persist for months or years and interfere with a person's ability to work and carry on a normal home life.

What can cause it?

▲ Various viruses: Epstein-Barr, HHV6, Coxsackie, hepatitis, influenza

▲ Work in an airtight office building loaded with pollutants: building materials which "outgas" chemical fumes like formaldehyde (lumber, wall board, carpet, foam rubber, paints, glues, waxes), tobacco smoke, perfumes, other cosmetics, floor cleaners, bathroom chemicals, copy papers, marking pencils, insecticides, and molds in the air conditioning system . . .

▲ Life in a home polluted with environmental chemicals: cigarette smoke, cosmetics, pesticides, laundry and bathroom chemicals, gas cooking stoves, freshly dry-cleaned clothes, and many of the same pollutants found in office buildings . . .

▲ Exposure to toxic chemicals in a factory . . .

▲ Acquisition of a parasitic infection . . .

▲ Life in a damp, moldy home . . .

▲ The insertion of mercury/amalgam dental fillings . . .

▲ A long term program of antibiotics . . .

According to Dr. Crook, CFS can be compared to a forest fire. It can start in many ways. Once it gets started, the immune system is weakened. And when that happens, look out! A vicious cycle can be set off that often goes something like this:

▲ infections develop

▲ broad spectrum antibiotics are often prescribed by doctors

▲ yeast infections result

▲ yeast overgrowth in the gut leads to diarrhea, constipation, abdominal pain, absorption of food allergens

▲ which leads to further immunosuppression
▲ which leads to more yeast infections
▲ and viral infections
▲ and bacterial infections
▲ and the potential growth of parasites

Eventually any and every part of the body can be affected. The individual can feel like he or she is coming apart at the seams! Fatigue, headaches, poor memory, inability to concentrate, abdominal pains, urinary problems, muscle pain, numbness, insomnia, palpitations of the heart, tingling in the arms and hands, cough, nasal congestion, and more![1]

Anyhow, Nancy's experience with EI and CFS all began as she sat in a warehouse full of beer. For fifteen years she worked as an executive secretary in the president's office of a large beer wholesaler in Dallas, Texas. Eight hours a day she sat behind a desk making sure things ran smoothly while most of the rest of the staff were out meeting clients and drumming up business. And eight hours a day for years she breathed in toxic fumes that eventually ruined her health.

"The product," she recalls, "was stored along the walls inside this huge warehouse that my office was in. Our trucks loaded and unloaded inside the warehouse without turning off their engines. Diesel fumes got into the air conditioning system, and I didn't know it. If I hadn't been as healthy as I was from the start, I could never have taken the insult to my body as long as I did."

For reasons unrelated to health, that office was eventually closed and Nancy was moved to another location. "It was the same thing," she says. "Just half a block away, our huge refrigeration trucks loaded and unloaded all day long without shutting off their engines. High, high pollution." And as she points out, "The air in Dallas is extremely polluted anyway. It's the sixth most polluted city in the U.S."

Seven or eight years into her fifteen-year stint with this company she began to get messages from her body that all was not well. First it was her eyesight. "All the vision from my left would move over to the front. If I was driving, everything on my far left would look like it was directly ahead." Her eye doctor knew it had something to do with chemical sensitivities, but he had no idea what to do about it.

Then came the gastrointestinal problems, accompanied by a host of expensive tests at Baylor University Hospital. "Seems like I was always at Baylor getting tested for something," Nancy remembers. "They passed me from one specialist to another, trying to figure out what was wrong with me, but never could."

Then came the joint pain. "I got so bad that I couldn't get out of bed and get to work on time. I had to set my alarm to ring an hour earlier, and I put blankets and pillows on the floor so I could roll out of bed in the morning, then crawl over to the chair. It was very, very, very painful. The doctors were giving me medicine for arthritis, but it was just making me all the more sick. They said I had a degeneration in my neck and sent me to physical therapy. The pain was excruciating, and of course physical therapy was not addressing the cause of my problems."

Nights would go by for Nancy without decent sleep. Hours were spent at Baylor looking for help and hope, to no avail. "My body was exploding with all these terrible things—sores in my mouth, excessive acid, diarrhea, and brain fog. My head wasn't working right, so I devised a way to keep my job without letting on that I wasn't really 'with it.' Anytime someone approached my desk, I'd look down at my paperwork and tell them I was too busy to stop and talk just then. I didn't want to have to try to be coherent. Truth was I wasn't. But I needed my job."

The doctors at Baylor had turned her every which way but loose, yet still had no idea what her problem was. "They'd given me *every* known test," says Nancy with more than a trace of disgust in her voice. "The last guy I saw there was the number-one doctor in charge. He said they were going to test me for a 'dread disease.' You know, in medical school that's the whole thrust of their training. They don't learn much about chronic degeneration like mine. The tests were exhaustive and took over a week."

Results? Nothing!

"At that point," admits Nancy, "I just stopped going to doctors. I threw away all the medicines they wanted me to take, and came up with my own plan. My body still hurt, but I found out about the technique of deep relaxation. I'd practice constructive meditation with God's guidance and would quiet my body into a state in which it could better tolerate the pain."

It was this "quiet time" that kept her going. "If I hadn't learned how to go off into my own little world and recuperate in silence, I just couldn't have made it," she says, her emotions evident.

EI can be a lonely place. She loved her church and she loved her friends there, but of course none of them understood what in the world was going on. They couldn't understand why she'd show up at church, then leave halfway through. They didn't realize that the new carpeting in the building was affecting her brain, sending her into "space city." Heck, Nancy didn't even know what was going on, much less explain it to others. All she was sure of was that in certain situations, her mind would go foggy, very foggy. Thoughts would be hard to put together. And what strength she had left in her aching body would simply leave her, like water being drained from a bathtub. Chronic fatigue dogged her days.

One day as she huddled in bed, perhaps trying to sleep off her tremendous fatigue, perhaps hiding from a world that had become a prison without bars, her doorbell rang. There stood four women, friends of her daughter, who were working on doctorate degrees in psychology at a nearby university. "Oh," they said, "we know what's happened to you."

"Well, I was so fatigued that I could hardly bear to try to talk to them, but I managed. They had a book with them that told all about chemical sensitivities and how it would make a person sick. One of their psych professors had a wife who worked in what she discovered was a 'sick building'—in other words, the air was full of toxic chemicals from paint, carpet, etc. The average medical types never could figure out what was wrong with her. She'd gone to doctor after doctor until finally discovering Dr. William J. Rea who runs the Environmental Health Clinic in Dallas. A surgeon by training, he had experienced what it meant to be environmentally ill when the chemicals he'd used for years in surgery took their toll on his own health and ability to function. "Anyhow, Dr. Rea told the professor what was wrong with his wife, and they began to collaborate. Rea needed psychological counseling for the many patients he was now helping deal with their own environmental illnesses. Their sense of hopelessness in the face of medical misunderstanding was a big issue. For his part, the professor went back to the university and said, 'I'll not teach psychology unless I'm allowed to teach one or more courses in environmental illness. The board agreed wholeheartedly, and that's the course these four women had been taking."

Armed with a compassion fueled by understanding, these women hovered over Nancy like a collective mother. Through their efforts and insistence, she finally made her first visit in several years to a medical doctor—but not just any medical doctor. This time it was someone who knew about environmental illness.

"I'll never forget my first visit with Dr. Rea," recalls Nancy. "He had me fill out all this paperwork, about an inch thick, asking questions about me that none of the other doctors had ever cared to ask. He looked through it all and said, 'Of course! Working around diesel trucks, that alone is going to make you sick.' And that's when he said those two key words concerning my future: *clean air.*"

But where? At work? No! In downtown Dallas? No! At home? No! In fact, after twenty years in the same duplex, she had been forced to move out for good. Huge ugly bugs had invaded her walls. The only pesticide she could tolerate was boric acid. The pesticide company agreed to use that, but just like the dentist, used something else instead. She was instantly sick and forced to move her life elsewhere, never to return.

Having by this time also lost her job with the beer warehouse, Nancy needed not only a place, but an income to keep body and soul together. She finally found a place that had what she needed—electric heat, no new paint, no new carpet, and no pesticides. It was a two-bedroom place, and for a source of income she began to house patients who came from around the world to see Dr. Rea at his clinic.

"They came from all over and stayed anywhere from three days to two weeks," she recalls. "One time I had three groups in there. They slept on the sofa, the floor, anywhere they could find space. There was an eye surgeon once who had gotten ill beyond belief from years of working around chemicals during surgery. He'd heard about me and called. He asked me to work for him. For the entirety of his stay I was his secretary, helper, and driver. I even washed his clothes. When he went to the clinic and saw the nutritionist, I'd take notes and give him a typewritten summary of the instructions. He had a hard time remembering anything because of the brain fog."

It was a great time for Nancy. She felt useful once again, and for a time her health seemed to be on the upswing. However, about five months into her lease she began to notice symptoms she'd never felt before. To her great disappointment she discovered that she was living next to a high-tension power line. Her symptoms were due to something called EMF's—electromagnetic fields. "The feeling of having all the energy drained out of my body was returning. I felt like I weighed 1,000 pounds. I had to move to another place."

Move she did, every six months for the next few years. "Landlords would promise me, 'No, we don't use pesticides.' Then I'd get up one morning a month or two later, and there would be a pesticide truck out on the street. I'd say, 'Hey, you promised me you didn't use pesticides.' 'Oh, well, we only do this every so often. It's perfectly safe.' It's very hard for people to understand that none means none. I developed a long history of moving."

In her search for clean air to feed her body, the EPA (Environmental Protection Agency) proved itself ineffective. Back when she still had her job, she'd called a top EPA guy in Dallas. "He listened as if he really cared," she recalls. "We had a long conversation. I told him I was sitting there in that office in downtown Dallas smoldering in pollution, getting sicker and sicker. Wasn't there something the EPA could do about it?"

Later that afternoon this guy's wife called. She said he'd come home for lunch, was telling her of Nancy's predicament, and couldn't finish because he started crying. "I couldn't tell this lady the truth," he'd told his wife. He could not openly agree with her about how bad her conditions were because of the politics that rule the EPA. He could've lost his job.

"We know exactly what you're going through," she'd told Nancy that day. "I was chemically exposed in my own job and my husband convinced me to quit when my health started to decline. Our prayers are with you."

Perhaps it was those prayers that brought Nancy to a significant decision. One day in the midst of the instability and chaos that her life had become, moving from one place to another, looking for a safe haven that would afford clean air, she woke up and said to herself, "This is not a life. I don't have to put up with this anymore. I must move away from Dallas."

A friend had mentioned how much better she always felt when visiting Colorado Springs. "The cleanest air in the U.S. is actually a tiny section of the country where Idaho, Utah, and Nevada all come together," Nancy points out, "but nobody lives there. Being a people person, I began to study wind flow patterns from the newspaper in Colorado Springs. I even contacted the air-quality control service in that city and got their advice. I eventually identified the best part of town for me to live in, and wound up buying a condo. To be relieved of the burden of being displaced and homeless all those years was a real blessing. It's such a comfort to know that I now have a place to lay my head; a safe haven for clean air that I have complete control over." (Of course, people still come down with EI and CFS even in Colorado Springs.)

Nancy Johnston had much more to tell me that day. She spoke of soldiers she'd met who had developed environmental illness from their service in Desert Storm. She'd befriended them at Dr. Rea's clinic. They told her how helpful his therapies were in removing the toxic chemicals that had been built up in their systems as a result of the oil wells being set on fire by the Iraqi's. She learned, to her amazement, that insurance companies and even the U.S. Army had refused to pay for these therapies.

She also told me stories about the doctors in Dallas who had little respect for Dr. Rea and his attempts to help people like her. "We all know about Dr. Rea," one Baylor doctor said to her, "and I can assure you that he is not going to meet your needs." And yet it was Dr. Rea who finally and, quite easily, diagnosed her problem after the Baylor doctors had taken thousands of dollars from her for tests that proved useless. They'd been looking for problems in all the wrong places. Dr. Rea had her keep a journal of when and where she felt sick. The mystery practically solved itself. In our age of high-tech medicine, the causes behind the illnesses that now plague us are often so profoundly simple, they're easily overlooked.

In the end, there's a lesson or two to be learned from Nancy's experience with EI. Lesson one actually applies to anybody battling any sort of disease. It's this: You're in charge. You're the boss in the business of winning back your health. Everyone else is just hired help. No one, absolutely no one, has the right to dictate to you what you should or shouldn't do—who you should or shouldn't consult. In fact, if you can't find health-care professionals who will work with you, call us here at *Health*Quarters and we'll see if we can't network you with more helpful individuals. (See page 229.)

Lesson two, environmental illness is a disease that will become more and more evident as our environment becomes more and more polluted. Those who are suffering now are like the little birds coal miners used to take down into mine shafts with them to help them detect dangerous gases. If the bird died, they'd be next if they didn't do something quick. Ladies and gentlemen, the "birds" are dying.

ANN THRELKELD

"If you just say you suffer from allergies, people understand," explains Ann Threlkeld. "But when you go beyond that, when you start listing all the things—the chemical exposures—that drain the energy right out of your body and make your brain go numb, then most people tend to look at you with a raised eyebrow."

She and husband, Bill, suffer from a condition known as environmental illness. In her own words, "a medically and socially unacceptable illness." Indeed, those who are battling EI are greatly misunderstood. Their physical suffering is often compounded by emotional wounds at the hands of unenlightened, perhaps even suspicious, friends and relatives.

Sunday mornings find Ann and Bill "in church" at home in front of the television. Large group meetings tend to be permeated with perfumes, colognes, fabric fumes, and a host of other air pollutants that can easily send their brains into such a fog, and their bodies into such collapse, that if they could even find the door to leave, they wouldn't have the strength to open it.

Although they feel isolated, at least they're in this battle together. "The divorce rate," according to Ann who has been diligently studying up on EI, "is 95 percent when one spouse develops the condition and the other doesn't."

It's interesting to note that women are much more likely to develop environmental sensitivities than men. It would seem that their biological makeup is naturally more sensitive to their surroundings. And perhaps its this greater sensitivity, expressed not only biologically but emotionally, that sheds light on why "well wives" tend to stand by their environmentally ill husbands much more readily than "well husbands" stand by their sick wives.

"When we first started noticing that something was really wrong with us, we had no idea what to call it," recalls Ann. "We were just confused. Bill could hardly make it into work, he was so mentally overwhelmed and physically exhausted. We finally got ourselves thoroughly checked out for everything under the sun—AIDS, lyme disease, hepatitis, you name it. The blood tests all came back clear, so the doctor just sort of wrote us off. He said, 'I'm sorry you've got this chronic fatigue thing going on, but your blood is just fine. I really don't know what to do for you. Don't come back unless things get worse.'"

They barely got home that day from the hospital before dropping into bed, exhausted. They knew something was wrong, terribly wrong. They also began to realize that the mainline medical community was not going to be much help.

"So many people out there are misunderstood and misdiagnosed by their doctors," explains Ann. "Most doctors don't know anything about EI. Ignorance breeds contempt. In other words, if they can't explain it, then they don't even think it exists—it's all psychological, in the head. You walk away from such a doctor with a false sense of guilt, like somehow you're to blame for being so silly or stupid as to think you had some sort of 'real' disease. Emotional pain is heaped upon the physical."

For the Threlkelds it took making contact with other EI sufferers to finally begin to put two and two together concerning their health problems. Once able to put a label on their trouble, finding professionals who could give them informed help was easier.

So what does a person need in order to win back their health from the clutches of extreme environmental sensitivities? You already know. Clean air.

Clean air, of course, is the primary tactic in the battle plan against EI. Clean air that will help to oxygenate body cells, fuel the body's process of throwing off toxic buildup, and fire up the immune system to provide better overall protection. That's the ultimate goal, a revived and revved-up immune system—an army God put into our bodies to fight our health wars. Also an army that can be subject to compromise if not properly maintained and looked after.

The flip side of getting clean air is "avoiding bad air." Besides getting out to where the air was clean and good, tracking down things in the home that needed to change was an important part of the overall strategy.

"We'd had a gas leak in our house," recalls Ann. "I could smell it, but the gas company could never find it. I'd had them out umpteen times over the last few years. Finally, while checking a valve in the back of the furnace, they found it. Our den is just off that furnace room. For thirteen years, Bill and I sat down there accumulating gas fumes in our bodies. I'm convinced that the toxic buildup from those fumes was part of why our immune systems became so compromised."

Another problem that may have had a role in their immune system overload had to do with the location of their bedroom—directly over the garage. "Bill still sleeps there," says Ann. "But we leave the car out in the driveway. The fumes from a car, even when it's turned off, can be amazing. And they filter up through the house."

As for her, she sleeps in a different room altogether. "Bill's allergic to the carbon in the air filter I need to use," she explains. "I've got a bedroom where I keep just my bed, a lamp, a table, and an air purifying mechanism with a three filter system. When you step from the hallway into my bedroom, it's like going from one world to another, as far as air quality. I try to stay in there ten hours a day. Of course, if the quality of air in our whole house was better, both of us would get better a whole lot quicker."

The Threlkeld's have been battling EI for over five years. "We're better," says Ann, "but we're not well. We want to sell our house and find a place to live that would be more conducive to our recovery. But it's been impossible so far to find a place that meets all our needs. One with electric heat, or at least the furnace outside the house. And it has to have wood or tile floors, no carpet. Carpet is a big offender as far as toxic fumes in the home. The synthetics it's made of can outgas for years, plus all the fumes from adhesives and the backing material. Besides all that, carpet collects a world of dust and dust mites, molds, and everything else people bring in on the bottoms of their shoes. People like us who have become extremely sensitive, just can't handle all that extra stuff!"

There is a man in nearby Denver, a professor of environmental sciences at a local university, who has patented a design for building toxic-free homes. Involved is a procedure for sealing off building products from outgasing into living space. Otherwise, the formaldehyde in construction materials, along with the various paints and adhesives that are normally used in building homes, form a toxic soup in the air. Ann and Bill are looking into the potential of having him build them a "safe" house of their own. Money, however, is an issue.

Besides clean air, an immune system enhancing diet is also of vital importance. Fruits, vegetables, and grains form the basis of such a menu. Sugars lower immune system response, and thus need to be avoided. Dairy products cause mucus buildup. Concentrated forms of protein, meat in particular, demand a great deal of energy from the body for digestion—energy needed for healing and rebuilding.

"We'd probably be further along than we are," admits Ann, "if we went at the diet with more discipline. But it's so hard when you're so tired and not feeling well. Many times, neither one of us feels like going into the kitchen to fix a health-promoting meal. So we do what's easy, we eat out. Sure, we try to pick the right places and eat the right things, but it's too easy to cheat. One step forward, three steps back. Seems like every day we're in a constant battle to do the right things to win back our health."

Summers find the Threlkeld's living in a small trailer they have parked in the nearby mountains of Colorado. Trailers are notorious for being made from toxic materials themselves, but as old as this one is, much of the outgasing has already occurred. With all the things they're exposed to in their home, their trailer represents a much cleaner environment.

"If we're back in the same house next fall when the furnace kicks in, we're going to have to do something," laments Ann. "I have to have clean air in the rooms I live in, or I'm never going to get completely well. I'm at a standstill right now. Even though I am better, I can easily get blown away by a dose of perfume or gas fumes or whatever."

Obviously, the crying need for Bill and Ann is to find or build a safe haven. Although they're not yet where they need to be, they have made progress.

MARGARET REED

The headline read, "Grad doesn't kid: Books sickening." What followed was a story about a student named Rita who was about to graduate from the University of California at Santa Barbara. The interesting thing was, she wasn't looking forward at all to holding her well-earned diploma in her soon to be graduated hands. Reason? A sensitivity to paper. Even a little bit of the stuff, the size of a diploma, was enough to make her sick. A whole book could put her to sleep—literally. In fact, Rita had become allergic to many things.

When asked to give her condition a label, she called it "immune disregulation and chemical susceptibility syndrome." That's a five-dollar name for being allergic to everything that goes along with this society. "Essentially, I'm sensitive to even low doses of toxic chemicals," she told the reporter. "That means paper and books, yes, but also toothpaste and carpet—just about everything with chemicals—even down to the colognes and perfumes fellow students are wearing."

So how does a person get that way? I asked that question of Margaret Reed, Rita's mother. For not only had Rita developed this condition, but so had Margaret and their other daughter, Cheryl.

Bottom line, it has to do with a weak or compromised immune system that can no longer protect the body. "When the immune system breaks down," says Margaret, "you get allergic to everything. Even food. Nutrients are no longer properly utilized. The whole body, including the central nervous system, gets messed up. One's health and body starts to fall apart.

"Symptoms will look different in different people," she points out. "A lot of times in men there will be heart attacks or lung problems. In women the symptoms are usually more diverse. Unless the woman has a doctor who knows the score, she's liable to be labeled as overly emotional, hysterical, or even crazy. The word *psychosomatic* has been used in countless doctors' offices around the country to describe this condition."

Were the Reed women born with weak immune systems, or did something happen to make them that way? Well, the answer is both. There was a genetic predisposition toward an underactive army of immune soldiers. From both sides of the family they had inherited propensity toward allergies and cancer. But a predisposition toward something doesn't mean it must happen. There were other factors, environmental influences, that pushed their bodies over the edge into the abyss of what has become labeled by those in the know as "immune dysfunction and multiple chemical sensitivity," or environmental illness for short.

Frequent illness plagued the family for years. In fact, months on end had been lost from the girls' high school careers due to sickness. The medical community was repeatedly consulted, and repeatedly unable to identify the reason or reasons behind their continual ill health. Finally, at the suggestion of some friends, the Reeds came into contact with a unique doctor who was specializing in environmental medicine. "After one visit," recalls Margaret, "we were convinced that we had been chemically injured."

A little environmental detective work bore this out. They discovered that a research lab near their home had admitted to dumping chemical pollutants into the ground water. They also learned that dry cleaning fluids had polluted a number of the drinking wells in and around their locality. Ah hah! Source one: water.

Source two? "We were living in Los Angeles, some of the worst air in the world."

Doctor's orders? Get clean air and clean water, and get it now! "One of the girls was already close to brain damage," recalls Margaret. "I needed to get them and myself out of LA fast."

Husband, Frank, had just joined the pastoral staff of a large church. It was agreed that he would hold down the homefront while Margaret shepherded Rita and Cheryl (then eighteen and twenty-one) out of LA to cleaner pastures in hopes that their immune systems could be restored. For just that purpose, Frank found and purchased a cabin in the remote mountains north of Santa Barbara. While mother and daughters set up camp in a tent-trailer parked nearby, Frank and a host of friends set about the task of renovating the cabin without the use of synthetic materials and chemicals.

In all about 250 people from their church got involved. Some provided all wool blankets, others 100 percent cotton sheets. These were an important part of recovery. One of the girls was extremely reactive to synthetic fabric. A man donated all the foil wall covering needed as a lining to keep the building materials from outgasing into their living space. Others donated glass and pewter cookware. Someone else sent eggs from their pesticide-free chickens.

For the whole summer, Margaret and the girls lived in the tent-trailer while Frank and friends made modifications to the cabin. Besides the foil on the walls, ceramic tile flooring needed to be put down. Fans were installed over both the stove and the refrigerator to vent fumes outside. Everything in the house needed to be electric. The television, because of outgasing from plastic parts, was placed in the fireplace behind glass.

With all the great help they got, their "safe haven" took shape. It would be home for the three of them for the better part of the next three years. Those first months were tortuous. One of the girls had become so allergic to food that the one last thing she could tolerate was cabbage. "Here we were in this cold cabin feeding her boiled cabbage for breakfast," recalls Margaret. "I don't know how many times I went to the farmer's market down in Santa Barbara wondering what I could find to feed her next, and some little old lady would be there who had grown some odd sort of organic tropical fruit in her yard. Foods you haven't eaten before are less likely to make you react. The big issue, of course, was that it had to be organically grown. No pesticides. We even ate some wild meat (legally captured, of course). When everything else is eliminated, you eat what you can tolerate."

Nutritional supplementation is also enormously important when you're suffering in such a condition. "The first line of defense that you work with is vitamin C," explains Margaret. "It's crucial in stopping allergic reactions, as well as helping to repair immune system damage. So you take huge doses of it, and if the person is allergic to citric based C, you go with tapioca-based or carrot-based."

Other important supplements included vitamins A and E, selenium (a mineral), plus acidophilus and bifidus to help combat yeast overgrowth in the colon.

And in addition to feeding the body, there was the issue of nurturing the soul. People who suffer from EI can become psychotic if isolated for too long. "It was important that Rita and Cheryl believed there would be life after this," says Margaret. "In the fall, they started back to school two days a week. It was traumatic. They had to go as handicapped students, air filters and book boxes in tow. (A book box is just that, a box with a glass top and gloves at the sides that allows a person to read the book inside without contact with pages.) People thought at first that they were a bit loony, but they both related well and made new friends."

If friends wanted to come to visit, and there were some, they'd have to start shampooing their hair with baking soda each day for several days before coming. Perfumes in hair take about three weeks to get rid of. Once they arrived, they'd have to put on a clean set of clothes and a cotton cap. Even after a quick trip into town to do a little shopping, Margaret would have to put on a change of clothes when she returned. "My clothing would be impregnated with gas fumes from the car," she explains. "It took some pretty heroic people to come visit us."

This story could get much longer and more involved, but the short version is that all three Reed women did eventually get better. They all still need to be careful about exposure to chemicals, but they have improved to the point of being able to make their lives among the general population once again.

As a result of their experiences, Cheryl is now in the process of getting her Ph.D. in behavorial medicine, specializing in neural toxicity. Margaret lectures to small groups and counsels individuals about how to make their lives more toxic-free. Rita, by the way, is on her way to a Ph.D. in English.

And where does Margaret start when she teaches others about toxic-free living? With the three most important things, of course. Clean air, clean water, and clean food.

ANN S.

Looking back on her life, Ann realizes now just how sensitive she was to hydrocarbon gas fumes as she was growing up. "We drove across the U.S. a couple of times when I was young," she recalls. "I was vomiting all the time. I'm sure now that it was the gasoline fumes. I also remember having to give up physics class in high school. I kept falling asleep. I realize now it was because of the Bunsen burner fumes."

Things started to come together in her realization not long ago when she found her health falling apart. "We were living in Italy. I got so weak and sick, I couldn't even hold a pencil. My mind would go blank, and my muscles weak. I'd lie in bed for days at a time, but my muscles would not recover. Doctors had no idea what was wrong with me."

Just down the road from their home was a factory. "We began to notice that I'd get better on weekends when the factory was closed, then sick again on Monday. We realized it was the factory emissions, remembering similar problems I'd had with fumes during my growing up years."

But that was only part of the puzzle for Ann. Another piece fell into place in the process of pursuing clean air. "We'd go over the border into Switzerland," she recalls, "and try to get up to an altitude where the air was cleaner. Sometimes I'd feel better, sometimes not. We wondered why."

Finally, she and her husband connected with the book *The Migraine Revolution*. It explained that some people have severe allergic reactions to things in their environment, like hydrocarbons in the air and even yeast in foods. Ah hah! That was why some trips to the high country weren't always beneficial. She'd sometimes take along sandwiches. The debilitating drain of energy was not only due to allergic response to gas fumes, but certain foods as well.

On the homefront, she turned off the gas in the kitchen and started cooking with electrical appliances. "Those hydrocarbons in the air lowered the energy in my whole body and were the prime mover in my health problems," she says. At the same time, Ann's sister, an M.D. back in Ohio, offered invaluable assistance. Major steps involved switching her to a different estrogen replacement formula (the previous one seemed to be helping to concentrate toxins in her cells); starting her on an intense program of mineral supplements to detoxify her body of heavy metals; instituting dietary changes and suggesting the use of beta-carotene, vitamins A, C, E, selenium, zinc, magnesium, etc., to protect against future exposure to hydrocarbons and food allergens.

Ann won back her health and strength gradually over the next months by eating a diet high in fresh fruits, salads, and grains. "I lost weight," she says, "and I felt much better. I stayed away from the stuff I realized I was allergic to, and my body really responded. I do have to watch my P's and Q's, however. If I eat a lot of bread with yeast or get around gas fumes too much, BINGO, I'm flat on my back in bed again."

Ann's husband tells the story of the two of them going to London to visit his mother. "We didn't realize what was happening to Ann at the time, but my mother had been cooking with her gas oven all day in preparation for our arrival. The windows had been shut. It wasn't more than half an hour after we had arrived before Ann was deathly ill. Now when we go to visit my mother, we ask her not to use her gas oven.

"There are a lot of people just like my wife who are waiting for the medical community to learn how to help them. Unfortunately, many physicians don't seem to know much about chronic fatigue or environmental illness. If we put into practice the ways of the ancient Chinese, there'd be a lot of motivated doctors. Back then, you didn't pay your doctor if you got sick, but only while you stayed healthy. It was his job to keep you well. A system like that would motivate doctors to figure out what's going on and help people get healthy."

QUOTES

"It is a rare person who can escape the adverse health effects of the 21st century. The average person is exposed to over 700 chemicals in city drinking water and over 500 chemicals in the home environment. The work environment and travel add even more."
—Sherry Rogers, M.D.
TOWNSEND LETTER FOR DOCTORS

"Next to nothing is currently known about the human toxic effects of almost 80% of the more than 48,000 chemicals listed by the United States Environmental Protection Agency. Fewer than 1,000 have been tested for immediate acute effects, and only about 500 have been tested for their ability to cause long-term health problems such as cancer, birth defects, and genetic changes. A National Research Council study found that complete health-hazard evaluations were available for only 10% of pesticides and 18% of drugs used in this country."
—Debra Lynn Dadd
NONTOXIC, NATURAL, AND EARTHWISE

"Because of the hidden nature of food and chemical allergies, the orthodox doctor usually does not diagnose the demonstrable cause of the illness. Despite the individual nature of the problem, he gives some mass-applicable remedy and does not deal with the specific needs of the patient. And because of the polysymptomatic nature of the illness, he often dismisses the patient's many and varied complaints as signs of hysteria, neurosis, or hypochondria."
—Theron G. Randolph, M.D.

AN ALTERNATIVE APPROACH TO ALLERGIES

FURTHER READING

An Alternative Approach to Allergies by Theron G. Randolph, M.D., and Ralph W. Moss, Ph.D. (New York: Bantam Books, 4th edition, 1987).

Chemical Exposures: Low Levels and High Stakes by Nicholas A. Ashford and Claudia S. Miller (New York: Van Nostrand Reinhold, 1991).

Chronic Fatigue Syndrome and the Yeast Connection by William G. Crook, M.D. (Jackson, TN: Professional Books, 1992).

Coping With Your Allergies by Natalie Golos and Frances Golos Golbitz (New York: Simon and Schuster, 1986), see chapter 5, "Ecological Mental Illness."

Healthy Homes in a Toxic World by Maury M. Breecher and Shirley Linde (New York: John Wiley and Sons, 1992).

The Nontoxic Home by Debra Lynn Dadd (New York: Jeremy P. Tarcher, 1986).

Nontoxic, Natural, and Earthwise by Debra Lynn Dadd (New York: Jeremy P. Tarcher/Perigee Books, 1990).

NOTE

1. William G. Crook, M.D., *Chronic Fatigue Syndrome and the Yeast Connection* (Jackson, TN: Professional Books, 1992), pages 21-32, 35.

10

NUTRITION AND LUPUS

INTRODUCTION TO LUPUS

Autoimmune diseases are those in which the body's own protective immune system fails to recognize friend from foe. Normally, the body would be able to distinguish "family" from foreign invader, however, something has happened to turn it against itself. In military jargon, the body has come under "friendly fire."

Rheumatoid arthritis and juvenile-onset diabetes are both part of this genre of diseases, two failings of the human system that we've already considered. Multiple sclerosis is yet another, coming up later in this book. And then there is lupus. Actually, there are two kinds of lupus—one that is systemic and affects the joints and organs, the other is a much less serious skin disease.

Systemic lupus is perhaps the most devastating of the autoimmune diseases, capable of reaching virtually all of the organs, sometimes one after the other, often with no warning at all. At least 80 percent of those who develop this nasty illness are women. There are many different treatments used in the world of medicine. The commonly used drugs, however, often bring with them an array of serious side effects.

Some people have discovered ways of successfully fighting

back against this terrible disease with nutrition and other nontoxic, non-drug means. In the pages that follow, you will meet three who are doing just that.

MICHELLE W.

At first it didn't seem terribly unusual to Michelle to be experiencing shooting pains in her fingers and knees. She was, after all, an interior decorator. A project she'd just completed involved hanging drapes. That could easily account for a little muscular discomfort, she figured. Those heavy wallpaper and fabric books she'd been lugging around could've been partly to blame, as well. Then too, arthritis ran in the family. Perhaps she was starting to develop just a touch of that. Maybe if she just ignored it, the pain would eventually go away.

"We went skiing soon after I completed the drapery job," Michelle recalls. "I did okay, but I still had the pain in my index finger. When we got home, it started in my back. I remember being jolted awake that night by a lightning bolt of pain that shot up my back. It didn't last long, so I just figured it was from the tow rope that had pulled us up the ski slopes."

The problem in her index finger, however, lingered. In fact, she began to notice that other fingers on the same hand were beginning to feel the same pain. One morning she woke up, and two of her fingers had become swollen for no apparent reason.

"I began to suspect at that point that this was something more than simple strain," she says.

Off to the emergency room she went, accompanied by her husband, Rick. The doctor checked her over and chalked it up to tendinitis, a simple inflammation. He gave her a prescription for anti-inflammatory drugs and suggested that if things didn't get better within seven to ten days that she get herself checked out again.

"Well, things didn't improve, so I went to see another doctor. I was in the midst of telling him my story, when one of his staff people interrupted and sort of matter-of-factly said, 'Sounds to me like lupus.' That made me angry. This wasn't lupus, this was tendinitis!"

Or was it?

Michelle didn't know much about systemic lupus, but she knew enough to know that she didn't want that to be her condition. She knew that lupus is an autoimmune disease, that you make yourself sick. One's own immune system begins to attack the body, rather than protect it. All the organs can be damaged—skin, kidneys, nervous system, lungs, heart. It's chronic, very degenerative, and has no cure—at least none that has been discovered yet.

"Lupus is a very difficult diagnosis," Michelle points out, "but after I realized what I had and how it showed itself, I began to remember symptoms. Several years back I'd had some problems with passing out. Also, whenever I'd get cold, my hand would not only turn blue, but I'd have terrible pain."

The doctors were recommending drugs. "I wasn't sure what to do," Michelle says. "I wanted to fight back against this disease, but I didn't want the side effects of the drugs."

At that point an acquaintance heard about the diagnosis and called. She got right to the point. "Michelle," she said, with an air of confidence, "there is another way. You don't have to put those toxic drugs into your body. There's another way to fight."

Michelle and Rick listened to what this woman had to say about fighting degenerative disease through nutrition. Later on that week they saw both a nutritionist and a rheumatologist on the same day. That night they sat down to compare approaches.

"The nutritionist was recommending natural products and was talking about detoxifying the body and rebuilding it through diet to function better," recalls Michelle. "On the other hand, the doctor was recommending drugs. Not only would they not be repairing my body to work better, they'd be toxic and would cause side effects. The best I could hope for would be a masking of the symptoms. And for how long? Who knew?"

This they did know, drugs weren't the answer for them. "We knew full well even as we walked out of the doctor's office that afternoon that we would not be following the medically correct model of treating this disease."

What happened next gave Michelle the motivation she would need to stick with the decision she'd made on treatment methods. The woman called back and invited her to a local support group of people in the area who were "into" alternative health-care methods. The guest speaker that night was a cancer conqueror.

"She'd been on her deathbed with cancer several years back," says Michelle, "and had been told by her doctors that she'd be dead within forty-eight hours. Yet here she was, telling her story of recovery, and thanking God for the wisdom she'd discovered concerning nutritional therapies for degenerative disease."

Rick had gone to the meeting, too. A peace settled into their hearts on the decision that nutrition and related nontoxic therapies were the way for them to go. "I hadn't been handed a death sentence like this lady," says Michelle, "but I had been told that I had a chronic degenerative disease that would just keep getting worse and worse. I figured, hey, if she could do it, so could I."

It was obvious from what the speaker had said that night that detoxifying the body was the vital first step to winning back one's health from the hands of a degenerative disease. Michelle made another appointment with the nutritionist, but even before that day rolled around, she'd already undergone three sessions with a colonic therapist. So important, in fact, is detoxing to the battle plan, that her nutritionist recommended that she continue weekly colonics, adding to that a series of three to five enemas a day, using a blend of distilled water, a bit of black strap molasses to keep her sugar level up, and hydrogen peroxide (3 percent solution) to help get oxygen into the colon and delivered to the rest of the system.

"My body began to throw off stuff that was unreal! Long strings of mucus began coming out of me. In the beginning, it looked just like we'd tossed angel hair pasta directly into the toilet. Then came the ropes, different sizes and shapes."

Along with cleaning house, a diet based primarily upon organic plant foods was employed with the goal of rebuilding the foundation of health. All meats were eliminated. Fruits, vegetables, and grains were maximized. Dairy products were greatly reduced.

"I know the problems other people have with dairy products," admits Michelle, "but I was instructed to eat a little cottage cheese or drink a little milk to help get amino acids into my system. We use raw milk, and I never drink over a cup a day. We will probably start making our own cottage cheese now that the government is allowing another synthetic hormone to be used in raising dairy cows."

Beverages included three ounces each morning of prune juice mixed with distilled water. She also consumed seven to nine glasses a day of freshly made vegetable juices—kale, spinach, and carrot. Freshly squeezed lemon with distilled water made for a refreshing lift when her glass wasn't filled with something else.

Concerning supplements, three times a day she'd take garlic, chromium, calcium, kelp (for iodine), aloe vera juice, gingko, etc. These things changed, of course, as she would periodically get checked by her nutritionist to see what sort of dietary supplementation her body required.

If all of this sounds like hard work, you're right! With all she had to do for herself, she had to get help with everything else she used to do. "I'd spend twelve to fifteen hours a day just working on my health—enemas, meals, supplements, and exercise. I worked out on the rebounder (small trampoline), rode the stationary bike, and walked every day regardless of how bad I felt. Even if I was dragging a leg."

But what about the pain? It had gotten pretty bad before she'd been diagnosed. After a couple of months into this program of nutritional and nontoxic therapies, it actually got worse. "It was so bad," recalls Michelle, "that it hurt even to have the bed sheets touch my body. It was a burning, ripping, tearing pain that would start in one muscle group, say the shoulder, and travel down my arm. Next day, it'd be in a new area. Each morning the pain was less intense, but by night it would become a gnawing and gnashing nightmare. It was so bad that I couldn't even crawl up the stairs to our bedroom. My husband literally had to push me up."

All the while, Michelle stuck with her decision to stay drug-free. She knew that the medications would only mask the symptoms, not deal with the causes. In the midst of her detoxifying and rebuilding process, she became aware through various natural health sources that mercury fillings in teeth can present a clear and present danger to a person's immune system. In fact, evidence continues to mount every day that dentistry plays a significant role in the health of the whole body, not just the mouth. If a person is allergic to metals in the teeth, naturally the immune system will be continually taxed to deal with this. Added to everything else the immune system should protect us from, you may have an overloaded and eventually an overwhelmed system on your hands. Even if a person is not allergic to mercury, it is nonetheless a toxic metal and emits toxic fumes. So say the professionals who are behind the growing movement to get rid of mercury in dentistry.

In an effort to do all she could to help reestablish the proper functioning of her immune system, Michelle had her fillings replaced with a nontoxic material.

As her body continued to clean out, heal, and rebuild, the pain gradually began to subside. "I don't really know how much removing my fillings helped," she admits, "but it's sure obvious that toxic metals in my mouth weren't doing me any good. As far as the colonics, enemas, and the diet, it's obvious what those things have done for me."

For over a year now Michelle has been free of pain and doing great. Is she cured? No. But it's obvious that she helped her body get to a point of control. The disease is no longer allowed to have its way with her. She's met the beast head on, not hidden from it behind drugs and medications that would in the end only make her more toxic.

What has she discovered through her experiences that she would like others to know?

"I want people to know that there is an alternative and that the alternative does work. Degenerative disease, no matter its name, is the result of a body that's just not working properly. Drugs don't help a body work better. They don't fix anything. They just mask the problem. The alternative to taking them is to go to work cleaning out and rebuilding the body. You can't effectively detoxify your body if you're taking in toxic medications."

ANGIE ROSS

While working on this section about lupus, I happened to come across this letter from an old friend of ours. With her permission, I share it with you.

"I went to college in 1976. By 1978, my health was failing. I was having blood clots lodging in different parts of my body. My platelet count was like that of a leukemia patient. I found myself very low on energy, had numerous rashes that the doctors said might never go away, and was so lightheaded I passed out several times. After much testing, it was determined that I had an autoimmune disease, Lupus E.

"I met and married my husband, Paul, and six months later found my body reacting negatively to the drugs I'd been prescribed. There was nothing more medical science could do for me, my doctors said. They went on to assure me that I would never be able to bear children, and in fact told me that I would be dead before I turned thirty.

"At that point, Kathy came into my life. She kept telling me about vitamins. I didn't think I could afford them. In fact, the doctors assured me that vitamins only give you expensive urine. However, I did finally give them a try for a month. I had nothing to lose.

"In that one month, my platelet count reached normal range. It hadn't been normal for years. We also got connected with a doctor who knew about nutrition. He took me off all the drugs and put me on a 'whole foods' diet, along with even more supplements. That doctor taught me about the negative effect that drugs and medications would have on my system.

"As a result of following his program of treatment and advice, I got stronger and healthier, and much more energetic. I had a normal healthy baby, and then several more. This in the face of assurances from those first doctors who said I'd never be able to have kids.

"I wish this was the end of the story, but in 1992 my strength started to slip again. Diet was no longer enough to keep me healthy. Something was attacking my body that diet alone could not address. To make a long story short, I had undergone dental work that year and had some cavities filled. The most commonly used substance, of course, is mercury. My body was reacting to it. It is, after all, a toxic metal.

"I felt much improved the day the first bunch of fillings were removed and replaced with a nontoxic, nonmetal material. I felt even better the day the second half of my mouth was done. Since I made that discovery and had my fillings replaced, I've had some days when my strength hasn't been the greatest, but I'm pleased to once again be gaining ground on my health.

"Dave and Anne, please ask your readers, regardless of the label given their health problems, to think back. Did their symptoms appear within six months after dental work? That was true for me when I first got sick and was diagnosed with Lupus E. It was true again when my restored health began to slip."

If I might add a moral to Angie's story, it is this: What you put into your mouth does affect your health, be it stuff you chew or stuff you chew with.

BETTY GRANT

"I've been dealing with lupus for over thirty years," says Betty Grant, "and I've counseled a lot of people. I tell them that I don't have a cure, but I can teach them what I've done to control the symptoms."

For Betty, it all began in 1962. She was then a young wife and mother, just thirty-two years old. "I'd been in bed the better part of seven years. The doctors who finally diagnosed me said that at my current rate of deterioration, I'd be dead within the year. Extreme muscle weaknesses, accompanied by a high fever (100 degrees), were unrelenting. No matter what the doctors did, no matter what drugs she took, the fever would not go down, nor would her energy level come up.

"I was taking both penicillin and cortisone, massive doses every day, for years. Back then, that was the best the doctors had to offer. Neither worked on the fever. My whole body was inflamed. I broke out in huge quarter-sized purple splotches. I remember one time being in the hospital and my young son coming to visit. He wouldn't even dare look at me. 'Why won't you look at your mama?' I asked him. He said, 'You sound like her, but you don't look like her.'"

Betty has since remarried, but life with her first husband found her packing up her kids and her drugs and heading south as her husband's work as an engineer took them to South America. Friends they made there brought her bark from a certain tree and had her boil it to make a tea.

"It's similar to the Pycnogenol they're now getting from the bark of trees in France," she explains. "That stuff is a powerful antioxidant, as apparently was the stuff in the tea I was learning to make. I drank it for several years, in fact the whole time we were in South America, and it did help to relieve the symptoms and bring down the fever."

When they finally moved back to the U.S., Betty found a doctor who knew something about nutrition. "He gave me shots of oxygen, which was a great help until the government decided to take it off the market. He also gave me megadoses of vitamins, in particular C. It is my opinion, based upon all the studying I've done and from the things I've experienced, that antioxidants are the key to fighting and winning against lupus—vitamins A, C, and E, along with trace minerals like selenium and zinc. These days, I can tell when I'm going downhill. When that happens, I simply increase my intake of the antioxidants—vitamin C, especially. It's very important. I don't go a day without it. I take at least eight to ten grams a day (8,000–10,000 mgs.). When I cut back, the old symptoms come back—arthritis, terrible headaches, systemic body pain.

"As far as diet goes to help control symptoms, I eat mainly lots of raw fruits and vegetables. And I've had muscle response testing with foods to see what I'm allergic to. My husband tests me several times a week on different things. As a guide, we use the book *Your Body Doesn't Lie* by John Diamond, M.D. I've had other kinds of allergy tests done by doctors. They have only served to confirm what muscle response testing, which is free and simple, had already told me."

According to Betty, exercise is also an important part of the lupus battle plan. "There are certain things I force myself to do every day, whether I feel like it or not. I have a rebounder, which is excellent for getting the lymph system going and the toxins flushed out. I jog in a swimming pool. And I ride a stationary bike. I can't do any of it for long periods. Perhaps ten to fifteen minutes at a time. I am, after all, sixty-five years old."

Comparing her experience with nutritional and nontoxic therapies to the experiences of others who stuck with the conventional route, Betty has this to say: "It seems like there's just no hope for them. The medicine is not curing them. Drugs don't cure chronic degeneration. And they're having toxic side effects. As for me, I finally chose to take myself off the drugs for a lot of reasons. I'd been having hallucinations, the drugs didn't reduce the fever, they didn't take away the pain. They just weren't helping me at all. I finally said, hey, this isn't working. Of course, my doctors got upset over my decision. But, it's my body, my choice.

"One of the fellows I counseled in the past stayed with the doctors and the drugs. He's not around anymore. It was his choice, his responsibility. I can tell people what I do, advise them, show them how I eat, what supplements I take. But it's up to them to choose what they want to do.

"A woman I was trying to help had gone through a divorce because of her illness. I told her about my success with diet and vitamins and gave her a bunch of my supplements. Two weeks later she brought them back. 'I don't think these are going to help me,' she said. I suggested that two weeks was not nearly long enough to influence her body chemistry and immune system. 'Well,' she said, 'I think some of them are making me sick.' I did muscle response testing on her. Everything seemed okay. It was obvious that emotionally, she just didn't want to go this route. I sat her down and told her that she needed to start taking personal responsibility for her own health, that doctors were not going to cure her. In fact, I told her that there's no cure, but lupus can be arrested and controlled. You can be in pretty good health if you follow certain guidelines. But she didn't really want to hear what I was saying. I'm sad to say I think she's dead now.

"It's just hard to convince people. We had a couple over the other night. We sat for over an hour and listened to their problems. Then I said, 'You know, it's not the doctors who are responsible for your health, it's you.' Well, sir, they didn't want to hear that. They were on prescription drugs and not sure about all this diet and supplement stuff. They'd heard all the propaganda about how vitamins are useless. But at the same time, they could see that the medical community was not really helping them. Things were getting worse."

When Betty talks with people about health issues, she's quick to recommend a book for everyone's personal health library. "It's called *Super Nutrition* by Richard Passwater, M.D. In the back he lists what we ought to be taking, far above the RDA. He also points out what we are not getting in our diets today.

"I do think," she concludes, "that poor eating habits are the basis for most people's problems these days. We don't feed our bodies properly, and thus become susceptible to all kinds of degenerative disease. The kind depends upon where we're weakest. I have come to the conclusion that the best therapy for most, if not all, of these illnesses is the same—nutrition and exercise."

QUOTES

"Lupus is another immune-deficient disease that is generally not being addressed successfully by the medical community. It responds well to diet and nutritional improvement."
—Linda Rector Page, Ph.D., N.D.
HEALTHY HEALING

"Diet in systemic lupus erythematosus, as in rheumatoid disease, is quite interesting. There is . . . evidence from animal studies that diets low in animal protein and high in plant and fish oils can reduce the severity of the disease."
—William E. Byrd, M.D.
THE LONG JOURNEY

"Mild cases of lupus respond well to supplements that build up the immune system. . . . A test for food allergies is helpful and often very revealing in cases of lupus."
—James F. Balch, M.D.
PRESCRIPTION FOR NUTRITIONAL HEALING

FURTHER READING

Healthy Healing by Linda Rector Page, Ph.D., N.D. (Sacramento, CA: Spilman Printing Co., 8th revised edition, 1990), page 207.

It's All in Your Head by Hal A. Huggins, D.D.S. (Garden City Park, NY: Avery Publishing Group, Inc., 1993).

Prescription for Nutritional Healing by James F. Balch, M.D., and Phyllis A. Balch, C.N.C. (Garden City Park, NY: Avery Publishing Group, Inc., 1990), pages 231-233.

11
NUTRITION AND MENTAL-EMOTIONAL DISTRESS

INTRODUCTION TO MENTAL-EMOTIONAL DISTRESS

We are biochemical organisms first and foremost. Some amino acids in the diet are transformed to neurotransmitters in the brain, so what goes on in our brains is very intimately influenced by what we put into our bodies. This should be no surprise, but a lot of professional people still don't see that. It's hard to believe that anyone would deny the effect of nutrients since we are totally dependent on them.[1]

CHERYL TOWNSLEY

The early Cheryl Townsley was in her own words "hard, abrupt, brusque, driven, and cold"—a woman out to conquer her way to the "top floor, corner office" of the corporate world.

Back when women weren't supposed to, Cheryl was pulling down a high "five-figure" salary and headed for six. Focused and fearless, she was out to take the business world by the horns and wrestle it to the ground. Although still in her twenties, she had the golden touch and knew how to use it.

"I had three degrees coming out of college. One was in teaching. The other two were a blend of business and computer science.

I began to climb the corporate ladder quickly. I knew computers inside and out—everything from programming to sales. A computer services company hired me to fly around the country as a national product manager. My personal and business schedules began to merge into one hectic day. I would have dry cleaning to pick up in one city, personal mail being sent to another, and sales appointments to keep in yet another. My house sitter kept my refrigerator stocked for my return, picked me up at the airport when I arrived home on hiatus, and returned me there when duty once again called. I loved the money and the travel. But even more, I loved getting results. The success of making the winning presentation and sealing the deal was intoxicating. In fact," she confesses, "it drove me."

Indeed, it was Cheryl's powerful drive to perform and produce that led not only to success in the business world but also to failure in relationships. In her wake she left behind the shattered remains of two failed marriages.

"As a Christian, I certainly didn't sanction divorce. But I also didn't see myself as the offending party."

It didn't dawn on her that maybe the problem was with her, not others. Success in the business world had blinded her to the truth about herself. That was about to change. At thirty years of age, married once more and pregnant, Cheryl was about to enter the roughest period of her life.

"I had moved on to starting my own consulting company. I completed several contracts, but the stress of satisfying those clients was growing. I'd also met, dated, and subsequently married Forest. Within five months I was pregnant. That was not part of my business plan.

"Because of complications with my pregnancy, I was put to bed for the last seven months. My physical health really began to deteriorate. Skin problems kept me itching constantly. My weight ballooned. And I had terrible fainting spells. I'd had certain physical problems throughout my life. I could never sweat before. My body just wouldn't. Even in PE at school I'd just turn red and get overheated, but never sweat. During my pregnancy I'd get overheated and faint."

As the months wore on, Cheryl's mental state began to hit the skids as well. Forest was unemployed. She couldn't work. Left without an income, they were forced to sell possessions in order to buy groceries.

"The stress and inactivity of those seven months ate away at my mental and emotional health. Here I was, this high-wire act—the belle of the board room—stuck in bed, fat and sick. I turned to food for comfort. It helped to chase away my feelings of being overwhelmed, inadequate, and out of control. Anything I craved, I ate. My diet consisted primarily of frozen Snickers bars, macaroni and cheese, and bacon sandwiches with mustard."

After Anna was born, Cheryl's health continued downhill. The weight she had gained stayed with her. Even though she tried to eat less, she gained more. Constipation was a constant companion. Skin problems worsened. The cares of life piled up heavier; the piles of unpaid bills, thicker. She was getting more and more edgy, more and more overwhelmed.

"Another attempt at launching my own business failed miserably. I had pulled together the investors and partners. As president, my role was to make it work. The pressure was overwhelming. We were under funded as a company, so there was tremendous urgency to get results quick or the whole thing would fall apart. At the same time, Forest was in the process of trying to get his own business up and running. The stress on our family was incredible."

As her business venture fell apart, Cheryl's health continued to decline. Deep, dark depression set in. Nothing was right. What she believed about herself, about God, about everything just didn't seem to work.

"I began to think through all the ways to kill myself. It had to be done in a way that Forest could still get the insurance money."

So much did she talk about being more valuable to the family dead than alive, that Forest took the unusual step of canceling the insurance policy, defusing her incentive to cash in her life.

One day, however, Cheryl hit rock bottom. Gathering all the pill bottles she could find in the house, she determined to put an end to her misery.

"When I tell it now," she laughs, "there is a bit of humor involved. I never did like to take pills. I'd never even taken an aspirin. And my throat is so small, I could take only one pill at a time. What I got down before I passed out that day, probably wasn't enough to kill me.

"I remember looking at myself in the mirror, seeing how ugly I'd become, and telling God that I just couldn't live like this anymore. I took the pills, one at a time and laid down on the bed. Just before losing consciousness, Forest's phone number flashed in my head. I wanted him to be the one to find me, so I called his office. When he got home he found me sprawled over the bed and called for help."

In the state of Colorado, it's a legal requirement that after an attempt at suicide, the individual must be seen by a psychiatrist. In Cheryl's case, the doctor wanted to medicate against mood swings. Having never been a "pill person," she declined.

"My health continued downhill. I became highly depressed, emotionally overwhelmed, and mentally muddled. None of my usual coping mechanisms worked. I no longer knew how to do anything. The thought of planning out my day was beyond me, really scary. Everything became slow motion. Somebody else had to watch after my child. I was incompetent. Every day when Forest would head to work, he'd make me promise that I'd be there when he returned. He knew that if I gave my word, I'd keep it and not try suicide again—at least not that day."

Forest's business had been "on the ropes" financially. It wasn't long before he had to close it down. Bankruptcy ensued. Then a foreclosure on their house. They lost it all, everything—health, wealth, and happiness.

"The three of us lived on $850 a month from unemployment," recalls Cheryl. "We were so broke that we prayed God would provide toilet paper."

About a year and a half after the suicide attempt, a friend told Cheryl about a local chiropractor-nutritionist she had been seeing for help with a detoxification program—cleaning out toxic buildup in the body at the cellular level.

"I took Forest with me. He was polite and asked all the questions. Truth was, I was pretty obnoxious about the whole thing because I expected to hear the same old mish-mash I'd heard from all the other doctors. At that point in my life, I was not into polite. That facade had been stripped away."

So, was the visit worth it?

"I was impressed! This guy thought he could help me and told me why in no uncertain terms. He addressed all my questions with answers that made sense. 'This is related to that . . . that's what causes this.' He was addressing things at a physical level that were having a cause-and-effect impact on my mental-emotional health. It certainly appealed to my sense of logic.

"The first step in the program was to come off all dietary supplements. That scared me. The supplements I was on gave me some good days in the midst of the bad. But it made sense that I needed to clean out before I could build back my health. It was rational to believe that any toxic buildup in my system would inhibit the level of nutrients I could absorb from supplements, even food. So, I took a leap of faith and began the program.

"My nutritionist had me keep a food diary, recording in it how my body responded. For the first month I ate nothing but fruits and vegetables. Then grains were added. Rice was first. About the third month, supplements were added to enhance the restoration and rebuilding process of my body.

"The food diary was a real eye-opener. Certain foods would instantly cause me to get angry. Sugar did that. If I ate a piece of dried fruit (highly concentrated sugar) or ate something with refined sugar in it, I would almost immediately feel my anger level rise and I'd become highly irritated. Fresh fruit, however, did not evoke the same response.

"Other foods would pull the plug on my energy. They'd make me feel like my mind was in slow motion, like I couldn't think straight. During that early cleansing period, grains were having that effect on me.

"It became obvious that fruits and vegetables were the best. As I got cleaner, the grains and dried fruits affected me less and less. They, too, were gradually added back in as an important part of my diet.

"Another part of this body cleansing involved a liver flush. I'd had an extremely painful gall bladder attack earlier that year. My nutritionist said this would help. For five days I consumed nothing but fresh, organic apple juice. I also took magnesium, a mineral supplement that helps to open the duct to the gall bladder and liver. Regular enemas were also part of the process. After five days, I drank half a cup of olive oil, followed by a citrus chaser (lemon or orange juice). Then I lay down on my right side for twenty minutes. The next morning I passed a handful of tiny gall stones. An ultrasound done by an M.D. confirmed that my once-crowded gall bladder was now clean. He was impressed. My mother'd had hers removed. Up until then, I'd been a likely candidate.

"Six months into this cleansing and rebuilding process, I'd lost all the extra weight I'd been carrying around since Anna's birth. After a year I felt like a new person, totally different in both behavior and ability to function. My energy level skyrocketed."

The Townsley's have certainly turned their lives around. Today Forest has a successful home mortgaging business. Cheryl is a sought after teacher-lecturer, publishes a newsletter called *Lifestyle for Health* (see page 231), has published three health and nutrition-oriented cookbooks and *Food Smart!* a book about how to make a transition from the standard American diet to a healthy one that works for the whole family (Piñon Press, 1994).

John Gleason

"Then he picked up a table lamp, threw it against the wall, and stormed out of the house," sobbed Linda Gleason as she painfully related the actions of her husband the previous evening. "He did finally come home several hours later, fell asleep on the couch, and stayed there most of the next day. I had to call his secretary for him and let her know he wouldn't be in. He wouldn't even rouse himself enough to use the phone. Just lay there watching soap operas. He's never watched soap operas before!"

Linda sat in the office of a trusted friend, a woman she'd gone to college with. Patricia, a pre-med major, had often asked for advice in money matters from Linda, a finance and accounting major. Now it was time for Patricia Brown, M.D., to return the favor.

"We'd just been talking about our finances, nothing big," continued Linda, pouring out her story on listening ears. "All of a sudden he erupted. He started yelling and screaming that I just didn't understand the pressures he was under. And then he tossed the lamp. He's never done anything like this before, Patricia. I just can't understand it. We've been happily married for twenty years. We've had disagreements now and then, but nothing like this."

Dr. Brown asked if Linda had noticed any other unusual changes in John's behavior.

"Well actually, now that I'm thinking about it, yes. I said that this was so unlike John to fly off the handle and then just lie around the house, but you know, other things have been different lately. Seems like it all started on a trip he recently took to South America."

John had been part of a group of men from their church who had gone to Chile to help build a school in a small village. John, a construction contractor, had been eagerly anticipating spearheading the project.

"He called home often," recalled Linda, "and I began to notice that he was not the jolly, happily involved man who had been looking forward to the trip. Now that they've all returned, some of the other men have told me that John just wasn't himself. He became more and more moody and irritable, the longer they were there. More than once he lost his temper with fellow workers. I know for a fact that John has never done that before. He's always, always been a very patient person."

Was she sure that this all seemed to begin in conjunction with the trip?

"Yes."

Did he drink only bottled water? Did he eat any of the locally grown produce?

"I know where you're headed with this, Pat," replied Linda. "No, he didn't get diarrhea. He did eat the local produce, they all did, but they were very careful to thoroughly wash it first. And they did drink only bottled water. They'd shipped their own supply from the States. We'd heard all the stories about parasites and bacteria you can pick up in other countries, so we took every precaution in sending them there. In fact, the minute John touched down in Chile, he began taking sulfa drugs to help protect against any bug or bacteria he might pick up. In fact, I think he's still taking small doses just to be sure, even though he's been home for a month."

That got the good doctor's attention. Sulpha drugs, huh? Antibacterial agents like sulpha drugs and antibiotics do kill off harmful bacteria and prevent its growth in the intestine, but they also kill off the good stuff as well. Healthy bacteria in the bowel, also referred to as intestinal flora, is important because it synthesizes a number of vitamins—things like riboflavin, biotin, and vitamin K—which are of great importance to the energy-producing activities of the tissues, particularly the nervous system.

"Studies have shown," continued Dr. Brown, "that abnormal psychological reactions can occur in people whose intestinal flora has been suppressed by drugs or even by a poor diet. Such reactions can include depression, anxiety, withdrawal, irritability, and a tendency to fly off the handle. The nervous system, including the brain, is just not getting enough of what it needs in order to function properly. In other words, Linda, what seems to be psychological in nature, may actually stem from a problem entirely chemical."

The next day Linda was back in the office with Dr. Brown. This time, John was at her side. Yes, he had been looking forward to the trip to Chile. But once he'd arrived, it was as if a deep depression started to come over him. Not right away, but within a week or so. "And the tiredness. I was tired all the time. And I found myself getting angry at the littlest things. I still do. I don't know what set me off the other night, but I just exploded."

Not only had John been continuing to take the sulfa drug, but he'd also become so depressed that food held no appeal. "That's right," interjected Linda. "Now that I think about it, you haven't been eating very well."

Blood was drawn. Tests were run. Discoveries were made. The drug had been a problem, for sure. It was the primary culprit in disrupting the health of his intestinal flora. The fact that his ensuing depression had left him without an appetite had compounded his problem. His blood-sugar level had dropped way below normal. Among the things that usually happen to a person in such a chronic condition when not enough glucose is available for the brain is a loss of emotional control. It can take many forms—simple nervousness, unexplained weeping and depression, even violent impulses like the immediate urge to smash something. And smash something, he did!

Following Dr. Brown's suggestions, John did three things that helped bring back the happy husband Linda had always known. First, he discontinued the drug. Second, he started to make himself eat. She recommended that he include plenty of starchy foods (potatoes, beans, pastas, cereals, breads). These were foods high in carbohydrates that would raise his blood-sugar level. Third, he was to take bifidous and acidophilus, two cultured products that help to restore good bacteria in the intestine.

Within days John Gleason was himself again. "It's an awful thing to have happen to you," he says. "That was my body, but that wasn't the real me. It's great to be back. I've learned a 3-D lesson. Drugs and Diet can lead to Depression."

JOHN AND TERI NIEDER'S SON

One of the Nieder children was a calm and agreeable sort. At least for the first eight days of his life. Day nine changed things. Dramatically!

That day he was returned to the hospital for his PKU test, a standard assessment done of all newborns to test for an inherited metabolic defect. They were required to hand him over to the doctors and wait in another room.

For a few hours after returning home, the child was quiet. "But then," recalls Teri, "he got real agitated. Suddenly we had a baby who just didn't want to sleep. He would maybe sleep an hour or an hour and a half in a twenty-four-hour period.

And so their lives were colored for the next four years. Did something happen in the hospital that day to send his system into high gear? Maybe, maybe not. All they knew for sure was that this was one very active kid.

"It was so bad," recalls Teri, "that at one point we took a

bed mattress and propped it up in the corner of our nursery. With pillows all around me, I'd just sit and hold my son all night long. I knew that even if I fell asleep and he fell out of my arms, he wouldn't fall far."

The grandparents were called upon for their expert advice. Was it normal for a kid to go without sleep for so long? This, they agreed, was unusual. They'd never seen anything like it before. He just didn't sleep.

At three weeks, the doctor wanted to get him started eating rice cereal. Not knowing better at the time, Teri followed the doctor's orders. The baby, however, got severely constipated. He'd go for ten days without a bowel movement.

"We'd call the doctor and he'd just say, 'Don't worry about it. It'll work its way out.' Meanwhile, we'd sit there and watch this little baby pushing and straining, turning red in the face. It was just awful. I finally decided to ignore what the doctor had said and put my son back on nothing but breast milk for the next nine months."

Did this experience with the rice cereal further compound the problems (later determined to be with his metabolic system) that were keeping him from sleep? Who knows. What they knew for sure, however, was that this kid slept many hours less than normal for his age, and his daytime behavior remained very active.

About the time their son turned four, a different doctor who was a friend of the family pushed Teri and John to consider putting their young son on Ritalin, an "amphetamine-like" drug that speeds up the body's central nervous system. For reasons not completely understood, it often calms hyperactivity.

"I'd been a school teacher and had seen firsthand the effect of the drug on children in the classroom," says Teri. "For some it seems to work okay. For others, however, it makes them lethargic, or even more hyper and emotional. Although we really didn't want to put our son on the stuff, we gave in and tried it for about two weeks. Our friend said we couldn't know for sure how it would affect him unless we did it for a full three weeks, but our boy developed severe insomnia, had huge circles under his eyes, and became very emotional. We decided then and there that there had to be a better way."

That's when the Environmental Health Center in Dallas, Texas, came into the picture. Teri had been reading books on food allergies. Dr. William Rea at the Center had written a couple she'd run across. They took their son to be tested, and to their surprise found that he was allergic to nearly everything they'd been feeding him. This despite the fact that for several years they'd been very careful about his diet, feeding him whole foods, avoiding processed things and sugary stuff.

"We'd known enough to remove the foods people are commonly allergic to—dairy, eggs, and wheat—but we had no idea that he was allergic to the otherwise good foods we kept feeding him, and that he enjoyed."

The doctors at the Center put him on a rotation diet. It began with an elimination of all the foods that caused him allergic reaction, whether strong or mild. Then slowly, over an extended period of time, the less reactive foods were added back one at a time. A diary was kept to note the foods eaten and response generated by his body. Various kinds of allergy shots were also administered. For him the program involved three years of careful diet control, with six months of shots.

"We saw real improvement in our son from the start," recalls Teri. "He became much calmer, a definite change in his demeanor. And he slept better. His digestion was also noticeably changed for the better, and his appetite picked up.

"We all adjusted our diets with him. You have to decide that this is what you're going to do, and stick with it. You're doing it for your child and for your family. It's not going to be easy for your child, nor is it going to be easy for you. But the benefits are far reaching."

What would she tell other parents who have children who display hyperactive behavior?

"We are very careful to avoid telling people not to use Ritalin. At the same time we encourage them to evaluate their child's diet. Eliminate the obvious things and see if that helps the behavior—things like sugar, artificial additives and preservatives, dairy products, wheat. Begin to read labels. I think it's too easy for people to cover up their poor eating habits with drugs."

ARLAND MARK STEWART

Arland Mark Stewart knows little about his six kids. Twenty-five years ago he began to suffer mental-health problems. Doctors called it a "manic-depressive" disorder. Deep, dark depressions would overtake him for days and weeks, shutting down life and shutting out his family. Financial problems mounted. Family life deteriorated. After nearly eight years of trying to cope, Mrs. Stewart filed for divorce and took the kids. Arland has had little contact with them since.

For years, his various doctors prescribed drugs to try to keep his depression in check. Somewhere along the line, he made the acquaintance of a psychiatrist who was using a new protocol—one developed by a Priscilla Slagle, M.D. This treatment was a blend of nutrients—amino acids, vitamins, and minerals—designed to provide the brain, and the whole metabolic system, with what it needs to function optimally. Arland made the switch.

Has he seen any difference?

"I used to experience huge, huge fatigue problems. I'd have to take a nap every day, I'd get so tired. But since using Dr. Slagle's program of nutrients, my health and energy levels have improved substantially. I'm hoping to soon be able to hold down a job and get off disability. Part of the reason is that those checks only go so far. I try to eat a health-promoting diet, but when the money runs out before the end of each month, I'm forced to eat whatever I can get.

Besides Dr. Slagle's nutrient program, Arland feeds himself lots of freshly prepared fruit and vegetable juices, plus a menu built primarily around organically grown produce. He's doing good things for his brain, and his brain is reciprocating the favor.

Special Note
The program developed by Priscilla Slagle, M.D., uses the following blend of nutrients as a basic treatment for people who suffer from depression: L-Tyrosine, L-Tryptophan (both amino acids),

vitamin B complex, vitamin C, and a multi-vitamin and mineral supplement. See her book *The Way Up from Down* for more details.

QUOTES

"In her practice, Dr. Priscilla Slagle, M.D. and Psychiatrist, uses supplemental amino acids, vitamins, and minerals to treat depression and other psychiatric disorders in her patients. She says nutrients are safer than conventional drug therapies, are preferable for long-term use, are virtually impossible to abuse, and provide additional benefits, such as increased energy. However, Dr. Slagle does not simply give patients megadoses of amino acids, vitamins, and minerals. She takes a measured and methodical approach that reviews a patient's history of symptoms, looks for signs of food allergies and side effects from drugs, and orders lab tests to establish baseline amino acid levels."

THE NUTRITION REPORTER
Jack Challem, Editor

"The answer to the question about how nutrition could possibly have anything to do with mental health is quite simple. What one eats, digests, and assimilates provides the energy-producing nutrients that the bloodstream carries to the brain. And any interference with the nutritional supply lines or with the energy-producing systems of the brain results in impaired functioning, which then may be called 'poor mental health.'"

—George Watson, Ph.D.
NUTRITION AND YOUR MIND

"When I investigated hyperactive children, I found that many of them were 'wild and crazy' because they were sensitive to dairy products. In some, the connection was easy to spot because they were pale, had dark circles under their eyes, and made snorting, throat-clearing noises as if they had some rubber bands hanging down their throats. The past history revealed colic as a baby, ear infections as a toddler, sometimes asthma as a complication of colds, and then the symptoms moved to bedwetting or nosebleeds. Headaches, constipation, sinus trouble, irritabili-

*ty and episodic violent behavior were often present, but we had
to remember to ask about them."*
—Lendon H. Smith, M.D.
DR. *LENDON SMITH'S LOW-STRESS DIET*

*"During the past few years, practitioners of environmental
medicine have begun to challenge the idea that psychosocial
factors are the prime source of psychotic disturbances. Instead,
these 'bioecologic psychiatrists' have demonstrated clear causal
connections between physiological problems and a broad spectrum of mental disturbances including schizophrenia. More
specifically, they have achieved marked success in treating mental illness as an effect of brain allergy, a widespread affliction
in which the central nervous system reacts adversely to foods,
chemicals, and inhalants."*
—Natalie Golos
COPING WITH YOUR ALLERGIES

*"Schizophrenia is an example of a disease that has been linked to
unmet, elevated nutrient needs. In one study, a group of schizo-
phrenics were found to have abnormal metabolism of vitamin C.
In another classic case, Mark Vonnegut, son of novelist Kurt
Vonnegut, experienced debilitating schizophrenia until Carl
Pfeiffer, M.D., Ph.D., found he had an unusually high need for
certain ingredients, including protein, vitamin B_6, and zinc. Only
weeks after Mark began following a nutrition program, his condi-
tion improved dramatically. He later graduated from Harvard
University medical school and is now a practicing physician."*
—Patrick Quillin, Ph.D., R.D.
HEALING NUTRIENTS

*"The combination of good natural foods plus the correct nutri-
tional supplements could eliminate most of the mental health
problems (as well as physical illness) and is inexpensive when
compared to drugs and doctor bills."*
—Carl C. Pfeiffer, Ph.D., M.D.
MENTAL AND ELEMENTAL NUTRIENTS

"A psychiatrist who refuses to try the methods of Orthomolecular Psychiatry (nutrition as related to mental health) in addition to his usual therapy in the treatment of his patients is failing in his duty as a physician."
—Linus Pauling, Ph.D.
AS QUOTED BY CARL C. PFEIFFER, PH.D., M.D.
IN *MENTAL AND ELEMENTAL NUTRIENTS*

FURTHER READING

An Alternative Approach to Allergies by Theron G. Randolph, M.D., and Ralph W. Moss, Ph.D. (New York: Bantam Books, 4th edition, 1987).

Coping With Your Allergies by Natalie Golos and Frances Golos Golbitz (New York: Simon and Schuster, Inc., revised edition, 1986), see chapter 5, "Ecological Mental Illness."

Food Smart! by Cheryl Townsley (Colorado Springs, CO: Piñon Press, 1994).

Healing Nutrients, by Patrick Quillin, Ph.D., R.D. (Chicago, IL: Contemporary Books, 1987).

Mental and Elemental Nutrients, by Carl C. Pfeiffer, Ph.D., M.D. (New Canaan, CT: Keats Publishing, Inc., 1975).

Nutrition and Your Mind by George Watson, Ph.D. (New York: Harper and Row, 1972).

The Way Up from Down by Priscilla Slagle, M.D. (New York: St. Martin's Paperbacks, updated edition, 1992).

12
NUTRITION AND MULTIPLE SCLEROSIS

INTRODUCTION TO MULTIPLE SCLEROSIS

Multiple Sclerosis (MS) is an autoimmune, degenerative disorder that affects the brain, spinal cord, and nervous system over a period of years. It is characterized by numerous lesions (areas of damage) on the nerve cells of the brain and/or spinal cord. Scar tissue replaces these lesions, causing the nerve cells to stop functioning. Each new attack (referred to as an exacerbation) has the potential of permanently robbing the individual of vital bodily functions. One attack may steal away vision; the next may plunder bladder control; a few months later, an arm or leg may go numb and lose its strength.

According to conventional medical wisdom, the attacks just keep coming, and the patient can only foresee getting worse and worse. Some, however, are fighting back successfully with nutrition.

DONNA HOMAN

"Your MRI is in the top one-third of the worst we've ever seen at this clinic," said the doctor. "You need to know that based on this test you can expect to be in a wheelchair in five years, be blind within eight, and probably dead in ten to twelve."

197

Donna Homan sat stunned. Was this really happening? Couldn't this please just be a nightmare that she'd wake up from soon? Tears flowed. As they did, husband Ralph put his arm around her shoulders in a way that said, "I'm with you in this. Count on me. Let's fight back."

For all intents and purposes, Donna was actually in pretty good shape—at least on the outside. She had, just that year, made a commitment to quit smoking. In the process she developed a disciplined program of rigorous exercise.

"My mother died of lupus when she was only thirty-three," she recalls. "Her birthday was May 9th. I don't make New Year's resolutions, but every year on May 9th I promise to work on something that I think my mother would want me to do for myself. I was thirty that year and had decided it was time to kick the habit. I'd been smoking since I was fifteen."

It was a habit, Donna discovered, that wasn't about to pack its bags without a fight.

"I found out that smoking can be the hardest addiction to quit. It was terrible! I know a friend who was able to quit doing drugs, but he still can't quit smoking. Anyhow, I became verbally abusive to everyone around me. My friends were all complaining about how awful I was to be with. My husband suggested I start going to the gym to take out my aggression and anger on the equipment rather than on him. 'It's steel,' he said. 'Equipment can take it. I'm just soft tissue.'

"Well, I got the message, so off I went. I'd sometimes end up in the gym twice a day just to alleviate the withdrawal symptoms. I found that I could put everything I had—all the anger, the anxiety . . . just everything—into that equipment."

Donna's newfound passion for exercise eventually paid handsome dividends. Besides kicking cigarettes, she dropped eighty pounds. New image in tow, she was looking forward to the future with enthusiasm. However, it was an enthusiasm that was about to be severely tested.

"One day after a strenuous workout on the stationery bike, I noticed that my left leg was feeling unusual, like a rubber band had been put around my upper thigh and another around my calf.

Everything in between felt funny. A diminished sensation. Well, I just thought it was a pinched nerve, so I didn't let it concern me much. Over the next few days I found myself sort of dragging that leg around with me, but I figured that if I kept working out the strange feeling would eventually go away. No pain, no gain."

Donna did keep up her rigorous exercise program, and sure enough, the strange sensations in the leg began to dissipate. But no sooner had they started to fade than something else began to happen.

"I noticed that I was feeling the same tingling and numbness in my upper right torso. I thought it odd, but again just chalked it up to a pinched nerve somewhere giving me trouble. The real shocker came when I woke up a few days later and realized that my eyes weren't working right. I could focus with one eye open, or the other, but they wouldn't work together. I figured I'd better go to a doctor to get myself checked out. That's when an MRI was done, and I found out that I had multiple sclerosis, MS.

"Needless to say, I was devastated. And I was scared. I just wanted to run back to where I'd grown up, and gather everyone around who cared about me. I was emotionally overwhelmed, and I went to get professional counseling. It wasn't any help at all. Thank goodness I have such a great husband. He was really positive and kept me motivated. He refused to accept as final what the doctors had said and launched us on an independent search to find out what we could do to beat this thing. We ended up reading all kinds of books on positive thinking. We reevaluated our priorities and asked our friends to be positive with us. Ralph told everyone who didn't have something positive to say to stay away."

Indeed, Ralph Homan is a fighter, an activist—a cause-oriented individual who enjoys going to bat against the opposition. It is not surprising that he belongs to an organization called Toastmasters. Here he is afforded regular opportunity to speak before captive audiences on issues that are close to his heart. And so, after making a presentation one day about their battle with MS, someone in the audience approached him with a bit of information that would change the direction of their battle plan forever.

Donna tells us, "This guy came up to my husband and said,

'Ralph, I grew up in Portland, Oregon. And the name in Portland is Dr. Roy Swank.'"

For years Roy Swank, M.D., has been working with MS patients. They come to see him from around the world. They come because they hear of his success with a special therapy. It's a therapy that doesn't require costly and toxic medicines, it doesn't require doctors and hospitals, it is easily administered in the kitchen of one's own home.

"His therapy has a 95 percent success rate for controlling symptoms in newly diagnosed MS patients," Donna points out. "A 95 percent reduction in both occurrence and severity of attacks. Even for people who have been progressing steadily downward and may already be wheelchair bound, this program can definitely stabilize their condition. They don't have to get worse. At almost any level people are in, they don't have to get any worse."

So what is this wonderfully successful therapy that every MS patient in the whole world ought to know about? In a word, *diet*.

"Every single patient that Dr. Swank has ever tested for MS has been found to be deficient in a certain blood protein, which should be there in healthy people. The role of this particular protein is to assimilate saturated fats. Dr. Swank says that if a person missing this protein eats the standard American diet—which is high in saturated fat—it clumps together blood cells, which in turn course through the arteries in the brain causing tiny hemorrhages. The areas where this bleeding touches the brain determine the location in the body where symptoms occur. Take the saturated fat out of the diet, and you can control the disease. It's not a cure, but it certainly is an effective way to control the disease."

The Swank diet, according to Donna, is really not all that hard to follow, once you get used to it. Especially if your option is taking Prednisone, the steroid drug commonly prescribed for people with MS.

"Prednisone is just terrible. You get mood swings like crazy. One day you might be higher than a kite; the next day real down. You just never know. And you get a false sense of energy, like you could go out and run the golf course. But it's really not physical energy—more of a mental thing. If you do go out and do something rigorous, the next thing you know you've crashed. And even though you're physically exhausted, the drug won't let you sleep."

On the Swank diet the MS warrior removes beef, eggs, butter, all dairy products—anything with saturated fat. The diet is built around foods from the plant kingdom, fruits and vegetables, with allowances for fish and the white meat of chicken and turkey if prepared without the skin. Three tablespoons of unsaturated oil are also included to help provide the body with fuel to produce energy.

"Nutrition has had a profound impact on my battle with MS," says Donna with conviction. "Five years ago they said by now I'd be in a wheelchair. I'd like to go back to that doctor and say, 'Look!'"

Donna has seen Dr. Swank twice. "After the second time, he said to me, 'Donna, you have the tools you need. You know what you have to do. You really don't need to come back to see me again.' I asked him if he thought I ought to find a neurologist. He said, 'No, all you really need is a qualified family doctor to check in with every now and then.'

"But what if somewhere along the road I have another attack? My original doctor told me that if I did he'd put me in the hospital for ten days and give me a bunch of drugs."

Dr. Swank's reply: "Well, you could go to that hospital, get those drugs, spend ten to twelve days there, cost your insurance company maybe thousands of dollars and see your premiums sky-rocket, and get all stressed out with doctors and nurses coming and going. Yes, your symptoms would probably eventually go away. Or if you have another bout—and this is what I would be inclined to tell you—you could just stay home and go to bed. Get rest. Feed yourself right. Have a few friends in from time to time who make you laugh. And eventually your symptoms will probably go away this way, too."

As Donna sees it, "Give me Swank's way, any day!"

There have been 172 articles published in medical journals about Dr. Swank's approach to treating MS. He's seen such good success that if you're diagnosed with the disease in England you're immediately put on the Swank diet. In the United States, it's another story.

"If you call the MS Society in the U.S.," says Donna, "they won't tell you about Dr. Swank or the low-fat diet. It's all drugs. It's as if they're censoring him. They used to help fund his research. No longer. The mainline medical community just doesn't seem to go for anything so simple and yet so effective as diet. The MS Society raises $70 million a year for research. And what are they researching? More drugs! In my opinion, that money is completely wasted. Mainline medicine needs to wake up to the importance of diet and nutrition.

"I told you about Ralph asking people to stay away if they didn't have anything positive to say to us. This was especially true when we started on the Swank diet. We just didn't need skeptics around. We almost lost several family members as a result. In particular was my uncle, who is also a physician. His whole thing was, 'Well, you know, they're just grasping at straws.' Now that five years have gone by, and he's seen what this change in diet has done for me, he now refers patients to the Swank diet himself. He says, 'Frankly, I'm embarrassed for my profession.' Those were the best words I could've heard from him."

Today the Homan home has become the informal headquarters in the Colorado Springs/Denver area for MS warriors using the Swank diet. Donna and Ralph are working hard to get the word out. You don't have to let MS have its way with you. You can fight back.

KATHY BREINER

Kathy Breiner has been in hand-to-hand combat with MS for fourteen years. For the first eleven her only weapon was Prednisone. To say that she considered the side effects of the drug annoying would be an understatement.

"The stuff's horrible!" she says with conviction. "I bloated up like a huge tomato. And I do mean huge! And the mood swings— I'm surprised that I'm still married. I'm surprised that my kids still live here. It was terrible on the whole family."

Not only that, but the drug didn't seem to work very well for her. Three years ago, Kathy was having real problems.

"Pain radiated from my lower back down through my pelvic area. I'd been told that there was no pain associated with MS.

I'd been told wrong. It was intense! Sometimes I couldn't even move, much less walk."

Through some mutual friends, Kathy was linked up with Donna Homan whom you've already met. Donna told her about her own amazing success on Dr. Swank's low-fat diet.

"Six weeks into the diet, the back pain was gone. I haven't had it since. It's been amazing. It went away, and I credit the diet with that. I also had the mercury fillings removed from my teeth. The larger medical community is just beginning to realize that mercury fillings can lead to all kinds of degenerative disorders, and in some cases, the onset of MS.

"I've stuck to the low-fat diet ever since. I haven't let up. Well, actually, I did let up once. I was testing my boundaries. I went out to dinner with my husband, and I had a piece of chocolate pie. Sure enough, the next day I couldn't walk. They say that stress can also bring on attacks. I must admit that I had a lot of stress going on in my life then, too. But thank goodness for what I've learned about controlling MS through diet."

It's obvious that Kathy feels like a caged bird set free. Others aren't so quick to join her flight.

"It feels wonderful not to have to be on the drugs. But when certain people ask me what I'm taking for my MS and I tell them, they look at me like I'm nuts. Just today I was talking with my gynecologist. She asked what I was doing, and I told her I was eating a low-fat diet and taking certain supplements. She gave me sort of a weird look and said, 'Okay, but what drugs are you taking, and what neurologist are you seeing?' The truth is I don't see a neurologist anymore. I've been lucky enough to find a local doctor who believes in Dr. Swank's diet."

Since opting for nutritional therapy, Kathy has lost fifty pounds. "It's not because I was purposefully trying," she says, "but because I was eating for health's sake."

The direction her diet now takes her is away from animal products and toward the garden. She eats only organically grown foods and avoids processed stuff. "I steer clear of everything that has hydrogenated or even partially hydrogenated oil in it. That's saturated fat. If you read the labels on processed foods, you'll find that most of them contain this stuff."

As far as dietary supplements, she's taking several, including vitamins C and E, magnesium, calcium, and flax seed oil.

The world of health science is not the world Kathy prefers. She's not the scientific type, not normally well versed on all the principles and properties of dietary chemistry against degenerative disease. "I'm not good at explaining why the diet works so well," she confesses. "But I can say this, it has worked for me."

BILL WATSON

When Bill Watson was thirty-seven, he began to experience mild double vision and problems keeping his balance. After about $25,000 in tests, doctors told him it was "all in his head." However, as a ten-year veteran of aerospace reentry physics, he knew it didn't take a rocket scientist to see that something was truly wrong with him.

"I went down to the MS society, and they checked me out. The problem is, there's no definitive test for MS. There are actually three levels they fit you into based upon the symptoms you exhibit—possible, probable, and confirmed. You have to have damage that shows up on a MRI in order to be considered confirmed. By that time it's obvious because you've got significant problems."

Finding himself with probable MS and not wanting to wait around until it confirmed itself, Bill began to read and study everything he could get his hands on that might help him to reverse his condition. His first discovery: the negative impact of stress.

"Stress can really bring it on. My first symptoms came during a period when I was more uptight than I'd ever been before in my life. My wife and I were having some real turmoil in our relationship. Eventually we got divorced. When my daughter was taken away from me, I had another significant attack. I'd lost my wife, my child, my house, my job, all my stuff."

As he continued to research, Bill came to a second conclusion.

"I read 110 books on all kinds of health issues and health practices, and in the end boiled them all down to one important thing. Nutrition. And in particular, the negative impact of sugar on the body. Everyone I'd ever met with MS was also struggling with a yeast overgrowth, also known as candida albicans. Sugar feeds this yeast, and the yeast can aggravate the symptoms of MS.

"As I did my research, I began to realize that sugar was also the trigger mechanism for the migraine headaches I'd experienced for twenty-five years. I began to remove all forms of sugar from my diet. My health improved dramatically. By sugar I mean all refined sugar, brown sugar, and even stuff like honey, molasses, and maple syrup. Sugar is sugar. They all bypass the digestive system and are absorbed directly into the bloodstream."

Eventually Bill got to the point where his exacerbations (attacks) were limited to only once a year; around Christmas time he'd gamble with a few cookies, and always come up a loser.

The final piece of Bill's battle gear came when he discovered the power of minerals. "For me, they've really helped to keep my MS in check. I now take massive doses of minerals, along with a host of other dietary supplements."

For all intents and purposes, Bill's battle plan seems to be working well for him. His mind is sharp and his body strong. He never did take drugs or follow conventional paths, but used his background as a scientist to learn how to be his own doctor.

"Originally it took up to five months to get my system back under control after an attack. After five years of studying, I learned how to get it under control in five weeks. After ten years I learned to put my symptoms into remission in just five days."

Quotes

"Dr. Swank has now treated several thousand MS patients with a lowfat diet . . . His results have met every challenge presented by the medical community, and are enormously superior to those achieved by any other known form of treatment to this otherwise crippling and usually fatal disease."

—John Robbins
Diet for a New America

"By any medical standard, his [Swank's] results have been remarkable."

—John A. McDougall, M.D.

"There have been two recent studies on the low fat/high polyunsaturated fat diet for MS. The first was done by Professor Roy Swank of the Oregon Health Sciences University in Portland, Oregon; the second was done by the Action for Research into Multiple Sclerosis (ARMS) Unit at the Central Middlesex Hospital, London. Both studies had the same broad conclusion—people with MS who stick steadfastly to a low fat diet do not get worse, whereas people who do not stick to it do get worse."

—Judy Graham, MS warrior
MULTIPLE SCLEROSIS: A SELF-HELP GUIDE TO ITS MANAGEMENT

"At the Informal Conference on Candida Albicans in July, 1982, the relationship of multiple sclerosis and other severe autoimmune diseases was discussed by the participants in attendance. Many physicians reported successful experiences in treating patients with these disorders with an anti-candida program. . . . Does candida cause multiple sclerosis, psoriasis, arthritis, schizophrenia and other devastating auto-immune disease? No, candida isn't the cause. Yet there's growing evidence, based on the clinical experience of many physicians, that the yeast organism, Candida albicans, is an important strand in the 'web' of causes of these and other diseases."

—William G. Crook, M.D.
THE YEAST CONNECTION

FURTHER READING

Diet for a New America by John Robbins (Walpole, NH: Stillpoint Publishing, 1987), see "Multiple Sclerosis," pages 279-282.

Don't Drink Your Milk! by Frank A. Oski, M.D. (Syracuse, NY: Mollica Press, Ltd., 1983), see pages 71, 74-75.

It's All in Your Head by Hal A. Huggins, D.D.S. (Garden City Park, NY: Avery Publishing Group, Inc., 1993).

Multiple Sclerosis: A Self-Help Guide to Its Management by Judy Graham (Rochester, VT: Healing Arts Press, 1989).

The Multiple Sclerosis Diet Book by Roy L. Swank, M.D., and Barbara Brewer Dugan (Garden City, NY: Doubleday and Co., 1987).

Special Diet Cookbooks; Multiple Sclerosis by Geraldine Fitzgerald and Fenella Briscoe (Wellingborough, Northamptonshire, England: Thorsons Publishers Limited, 1989).

The Yeast Connection by William G. Crook, M.D. (Jackson, TN: Professional Books, 1983), see "Does Candida Cause Multiple Sclerosis, Psoriasis, Arthritis or Schizophrenia?" pages 218-228.

13
NUTRITION AND OTHER COMMON AILMENTS

INTRODUCTION

What do you own that is a marvel of mechanical engineering, gets you from place to place, and would cost you more than "an arm and a leg" to replace? If you answered *a body*, you'd be right. I'm on solid ground when I contend that we've all got one on our list of personal possessions. And just like the cars many of us also own, our bodies need special care. What we put into our "tanks" is of utmost importance. It is my hope that if you haven't already, you're moving quickly toward the conclusion that nutrition is of fundamental importance to human health and well-being.

In harvesting material for this book, some of the stories we uncovered didn't fit into our prearranged menu. Although these individual "peas" have no preestablished "pod" to draw them together as a unit, they nonetheless contribute nicely to the over-all feast. I think you will find the following stories further evidence of the vital link between nutrition and health.

PHIL M., M.D.
Cataracts
"And this worked for your wife?" I asked Phil, a retired medical doctor.

"Oh, yes, indeed!" came his emphatic reply. "She was actually anticipating the need for cataract surgery. Her eye doctor had fit her with stronger and stronger glasses, but her cataracts were getting to the point where light wouldn't go through them much any more."

A cataract is a clouded condition in the lens of the eye, resulting in blurred and dim vision. It happens slowly. In the early stages, difficulty in seeing may be helped by eyeglasses. As the condition worsens, the power of the glasses is increased. Conventional medicine says that eventually surgery is needed for any hope of seeing. Mrs. M was just about there.

"She'd gotten to the point where night driving was impossible. In fact, even in daylight she was having trouble reading road signs. So that's when we saw Dr. Todd.

"We'd read about his work with cataracts in Jane Heimlich's book *What Your Doctor Won't Tell You*. We went to see him, and my wife started taking his formula of vitamin and mineral supplementation, which includes a special blend of several of the trace minerals. Anyhow, within three months she was much improved. She could read two lines lower on the eye chart and has been able to go back to a less powerful eyeglass prescription. The cataracts are not completely gone yet, but they're a whole lot better."

That's wonderful! A nutritional therapy that helps cataracts. Have others been helped, too?

"Well, people are coming to see Dr. Todd from all over the east coast. And he's not the only doctor doing this. There are others. We've heard many stories of people getting better without surgery. Dr. Todd claims that this sort of vitamin and mineral therapy will help the kind of cataracts that older people like my wife get. In fact, we have a seventy-seven-year-old friend with macular degeneration, a condition that causes a blind spot to appear when the individual looks directly at something. Her eye doctor had nothing to offer. When she asked about vitamin and mineral therapy, he pooh-poohed it. Well, she started taking Dr. Todd's formula anyway, and she's much improved. Just like my wife, she's been able to switch back to less powerful eyeglasses."

I asked Dr. M why he thought information about this sort of help for people suffering from cataracts hasn't received more widespread coverage. His answer was interesting, coming from someone with M.D. after his name.

"Dr. Todd is an eye surgeon who came up with a nonsurgical, cost-effective way to help people with cataracts. . . . Well, that threatens to reduce a very lucrative industry. A doctor who does cataract surgery can make $2000 an eye, and can average twenty eyes a week. That's two million dollars a year just for cataracts, not including whatever else he does!"

Bottom line: Money talks. Livelihoods could be at stake.

TRACY KEHRER, R.N.

Menstrual Cramps and Morning Sickness
Tracy Kehrer stood in her kitchen all afternoon riveted to the pages of a book she could not put down. "I picked it up and read it from cover to cover, and just let my house go to pot," she admits. "It stirred me so much."

Anne's triumph over cancer, documented in our book *A Cancer Battle Plan*, brought back for Tracy vivid memories of hospitalized cancer patients she'd cared for as a registered nurse. There, too, lingered the heart-wrenching memories of her grandmother's recent agonizing death from the dread disease.

"Anne's experience forced me to recognize the credibility of naturopathic medicine as a viable alternative to today's traditional medical practices. I began to see with new eyes that modern medicine is wonderful for crisis intervention, but for prevention and for maintenance of health, it's just terrible."

You don't often hear such an appraisal from people trained to administer the drugs and surgery of modern medical practice. Granted, we do have the best medical care in the entire world if you've been shot, hit by a car, or fallen off a ladder. But if you have cancer or any of a number of other chronic degenerative diseases, the statistics are not encouraging. One wonders if our modern health-care system is just not designed to treat such conditions effectively. Instead of helping to clean out, restore, and regenerate the body's God-given protective systems, we are invited to cut, burn, and poison—treating symptoms rather than causes. And if your condition is chronic, but not life threatening, you'll just get drugged to mask the symptoms.

Tracy's concern was one of the latter—chronic, but not life threatening. She'd had three kids, and with each pregnancy she suffered more and more intensely from morning sickness. Acute nausea and vomiting haunted her days. Occasionally it got so bad that hospitalization was required. "Many women experience nausea during their first trimester. Mine was extreme! For the first four or five months I would put up baby gates around the house and just let my other babies play while I literally crawled from room to room."

In the midst of vomiting with her third pregnancy, Tracy read something that suggested fasting as a possible treatment for morning sickness. "I tried it. I fasted for two days, threw up all the first day, but for the next four felt good. Problem was, it wasn't a lasting cure. The nausea returned."

Even so, she says, the groundwork was being laid for her openness to the principle of detoxification introduced to her through *A Cancer Battle Plan*. Other sources that spoke about natural healing and the need to clean out our bodies found their way into her life. She discovered a copy of a magazine called *Gentle Spirit*, aimed at encouraging "stay-at-home" mothers. "I found intriguing articles by Christopher Deatherage, a naturopathic physician, and Carol Cahours, a midwife and 'backyard herbalist.' They both emphasized vegetarian diets and herbal treatments for various conditions. Even more fascinating were the personal successes of those who followed their recommendations." Again, more groundwork was being laid in her thinking.

"At the time when I read *A Cancer Battle Plan*, my husband and I were considering whether or not we wanted to have another child. We'd always wanted a big family, but I knew I couldn't go through more of those horrible months. I just couldn't! Yet we both felt an assurance that I should get pregnant again." This time, she hoped, things would be different.

"With my husband's full support, I launched myself on an adventure of detoxification. Taking Anne's advice from *A Cancer*

Battle Plan, I sought out the supervision of a professional who had the clinical experience in nutrition and detoxification that I lacked, even as an R.N. Through a friend, I wound up working with Dr. Peter Petropulos, both a chiropractor and naturopathic physician. First step, 'the Daniel diet.'"

It's called that because it's based on the food Daniel of the Bible asked for while in preparation for service to King Nebuchadnezzar of ancient Babylon. The king wanted Daniel to eat a bunch of rich foods, the king's own fare, but Daniel begged off. Some say it was for spiritual reasons. The king's food had been used in worshiping an idol. Daniel wanted no part of that. Others say it was because some of what the king was offering was pork, a food forbidden for Jews in the Levitical writings. Bottom line, one reason that seems to make sense from the text is that Daniel simply knew that the kings' rich foods would lead him down the path of poor health. After a ten-day diet of nothing but water and vegetables, Daniel and three of his buddies, who had also decided to just say no, looked healthier and better nourished than the others who had feasted on what was supplied directly from the king's table.

Anyhow, a repeat of what Daniel had done was what the good doctor suggested as a first step for Tracy. "The whole program included three phases. Phase one was called the immune sensitization (IS) phase and lasted for seven days. I ate only fruits and vegetables, either raw or lightly steamed. Two days in I got dizzy, lethargic, and chilled. That night I had persistent hiccups and a headache, but by day three these responses to my body's detoxifying process had stopped."

Only hypo-allergenic foods were allowed that first week, the kind of stuff most people are not allergic to. Food allergies are a bigger problem with most of us than we think. And you can't detoxify your system if you're feeding it stuff that is causing mucus buildup from an allergic response. The list of fresh produce Tracy ate was as follows: all green leafy stuff (except iceberg lettuce), artichokes, asparagus, beets, broccoli, Brussels sprouts, carrots, cauliflower, cucumbers, dandelion greens, dicon radishes, endive, green beans, ginger, Jerusalem artichokes, kale, kohlrabi,okra, parsley, parsnips, pumpkins, radishes, rutabaga, spinach, squash (any variety), Swiss chard, and turnips. Interestingly enough, no onions, potatoes, or garlic. Why not? These are not considered hypo-allergenic. In other words, they do cause allergic responses in certain people.

"In the weeks that followed, phase two found me reintroducing different foods into my diet, one at a time to see what sort of response they would cause in my body. This included things like rice, various kinds of beans, and fruits and vegetables not on the hypo-allergenic list. At Dr. Petropulos' recommendation, I waited about four months before reintroducing the five most common allergens—eggs, dairy products, soybeans and soy products, corn and corn products, and gluten protein found in wheat, oats, rye, barley, and their products. These, in fact, were among the last foods I reintroduced prior to the third and last phase, which is the stabilization and maintenance (SAM) phase. I started that after all my detoxifying was done."

And detoxify she did. At the same time that she was reintroducing foods, she was also taking a mixture of herbs formulated to help flush her system. Gas became a problem, a signal to Dr. Petropulos that it was time for the liver–gall-bladder flush.

"This procedure," explains Tracy, "is primarily intended to cleanse the gallbladder and biliary ductal system. I had no idea what it would do for my liver, and I confess that it seemed very radical to me. But then again, I was willing to give it a try."

Her first liver flush began five weeks after beginning the Daniel diet. Along with her newly tailored diet, she drank two quarts a day of freshly squeezed apple juice mixed with thirty drops of orthophosphoric acid (a phosphorous supplement the doctor recommended). The agents in apple juice help to hyper-stimulate the gallbladder. Each day she also gave herself an enema, two tablespoons of catnip steeped in one and a half quarts of water, cooled, of course, before insertion. Coffee enemas are popular for this purpose, but Dr. Petropulos felt that might be too harsh for Tracy's system.

When day six rolled around, the game plan shifted. Two hours after lunch she drank three ounces of warm water with two tablespoons of Epsom salts dissolved in it. Two hours after that, she gave herself a one-quart enema containing a fourth cup of Epsom salts. An hour after that, she downed another tablespoon of Epsom salts in three ounces of water. Citrus fruit was the food of choice for dinner, then three-fourths cup of extra virgin olive oil just before bed.

"Then I was to immediately lie on my right side with my right knee drawn up to my chin, and hold it there for at least thirty minutes. This encourages the oil to drain from the stomach, helping the contents of the gallbladder and liver to move into the small intestine. Next morning, another Epsom salts enema, plus downing another tablespoon of the stuff in three ounces of water."

The success of the flush was an unexpected surprise for Tracy. "The next morning I started to pass what I initially thought was feces. But then I remembered that I had already passed all the contents of my intestines the prior evening. Upon closer examination, I realized that these stools were the kelly green to olive drab color of bile, and they were actually gallstones that had been softened by the oil and purged from my gallbladder. I had no idea that at age twenty-eight I had gallstones. I was further shocked that I passed a cup and a half, some over an inch in diameter."

By the way, in the midst of all this detoxifying Tracy experienced unexpected beneficial side effects. Although she admitted to eating three times as much as she used to, she lost ten pounds. Her energy level skyrocketed. "I had more drive and stronger immunity than I'd experienced in months." And she had periods without pain. That's right, without pain! "In the past, I'd always have a headache the night before I started my period, so I'd take some ibuprofen. However, once I began this detox program, I had no headaches and no cramping throughout each of my monthly cycles."

Tracy had met with success at every turn. Even so, there was still more flushing to be done. Three weeks later, on her doctor's recommendation, she did another. Then three weeks after that, yet another. Three liver flushes in all. And the final tally in gallstones? Almost three cups.

"The impact of realizing how sick and sluggish my liver and gallbladder were pulled the pieces of the puzzle together in regards to my struggle with morning sickness. During the early weeks of pregnancy, the liver is called upon to change a host of pregnancy related hormones into a form that can be eliminated through the kidneys. That, of course, is why a urine test shows whether you're pregnant. Anyhow, the liver is being overloaded with toxic waste during this time. If it's already sluggish, so sluggish as to allow bile to turn into gallstones, this overload simply sends the liver into shock. Since it is the detoxifying center of the body, the whole system becomes toxic. A condition develops where all food is perceived by the body as poison, it simply can't handle it. Nothing smells good, nothing tastes good. Bottom line, a constant state of what has come to be called morning sickness."

And so, the adventure Tracy had launched herself on had now been completed. A clean body and a ready heart. Time to get pregnant again. And that's just what she did.

"Shortly after I performed the third flush, our third child was weaned, and I was blessed by our fourth conception. I am right now sixteen weeks along, and I have had no vomiting at all. Although my appetite has decreased, I am not chronically nauseous. In fact, I only feel an occasionally passing flash of queasiness if I wait too long to eat or get too tired without realizing it. I am more tired than I expected to be, but I am not experiencing the severe, chronic exhaustion I usually felt. In fact, my energy level is increasing more with each passing day. I am not back to my post-detoxification levels of high appetite, energy, and immunity, however I feel vastly different from my other three pregnancies. I'm awed by the contrast."

TRISH HAZZARD
Wilson's Syndrome
Symptoms can include a blend of the following: fatigue, headaches (including migraines), PMS, irritability, dry hair, hair loss, decreased memory and concentration, insomnia and narcolepsy, anxiety, panic attacks, depression, heat and/or cold intolerance, cold hands and feet, fluid retention, inappropriate weight gain, constipation, irritable bowel syndrome, acid indigestion, allergies, asthma, dry skin, itchiness, hives, psoriasis, changes in skin and hair pigmentation, flushing, unhealthy nails, decreased motivation and ambition, inhibited sexual development, decreased sex

drive and anhedonia (capacity to enjoy life), irregular periods and menstrual cramps, infertility, decreased self-esteem, decreased wound healing, increased skin infections and acne, recurrent infections, hemorrhoids, hypoglycemia, low blood pressure, lightheadedness, food cravings, food intolerances, increased post-prandial response (exaggerated drowsiness afer eating), elevated cholesterol levels, dry eyes and blurred vision, carpal tunnel syndrome, arthritis and muscular/joint aches, musculoskeletal strains, increased bruising, tinnitus (ringing in the ears), abnormal throat and swallowing sensations, canker sores, bad breath, lack of coordination, sweating abnormalities, increased susceptibility to substance abuse.

Wilson's syndrome (WS). That's what it's been dubbed in medical circles. It gets its name after Dennis Wilson, M.D., primary expert on this malady of the human frame.

So what is Wilson's syndrome? In simple terms, it's a condition in which the body has gone into hibernation. The whole metabolic system has been slowed way down. Metabolism, of course, is the sum total of all the chemical reactions in the body. Without these, there is no life. Under conditions of impaired metabolism a smorgasbord of symptoms arise, which while not immediately life threatening, are evidence that the body is caught in a downward spiral toward greater and greater disrepair. It very well could be that many of the degenerative diseases that plague modern-day America find their genesis in a body first weakened by Wilson's syndrome.

So what is it that actually serves to put the brakes on the metabolic rate of the body?In a domino-like progression, indicative of the synergy that has been designed into the human body, each part of our metabolic system depends upon all the others in order to function. Following metabolic slow-down back to its source, metabolism depends upon the proper functioning of the body's enzymes. Enzymes are the catalysts for all the chemical reactions in the body. They are to the human frame what spark plugs are to a car. If a car's spark plugs are not working well, it won't run well regardless of the quality of fuel in its tank. Likewise, if a body's enzyme power has been compromised, it won't work well

regardless of the health-promoting qualities of the food eaten.
For enzymes to function optimally, body temperature must be
98.6. Any lower, and the enzymes don't work as well. It's like tuning a radio. If the station is found on the dial at 98.6, then optimal performance is found by tuning into that exact point. Any vari-
ance leads to diminished quality. The same is true in the case of
enzymes. Unless the body thermostat is set at 98.6, enzyme performance is compromised.

The regulation of body temperature is a major function of the
thyroid hormone system. If not enough of the hormone liothyro-
nine (also called T3) is produced in the body, temperature will be
low, thus affecting the performance of enzymes. And what affects
the production of T3 in the body? Various kinds of stress.

Our bodies have two modes of operation—a productivity mode
and a conservation mode—Dr. Wilson points out: "The body enters
into the conservation mode under conditions that threaten the survival and/or physical, mental, emotional resources of the body."[1]
Such stressors might come in the form of illness, surgery or acci-
dents, giving birth, getting divorced, experiencing the death of a
loved one, enduring job or family stress, being abused or molested
as a child, starvation (not common in the U.S. except for severe
dieting and anorexia), etc.

The chain, then, looks like this:

various stressors on the body
can lead to impaired thyroid hormone system (and
    under-production of T3),
which can lead to low body temperature,
which can lead to impaired enzyme performance,
which can lead to impaired metabolism,
which can lead to the host of symptoms listed above, if the
    body stays in the conservation mode for an extended
    period of time.

"When the stressful conditions have passed," explains Dr. Wilson,
"the body is supposed to return to the productivity mode; but in
Wilson's syndrome it doesn't, leaving people to suffer with frustrating

and often debilitating complaints long after the stress has passed." He goes on to explain that thyroid blood tests often appear in "normal range." The most accurate indicator of WS is low body temperature. Proper nutrition, activity, and sleep can sometimes improve the system, but are often insufficient to correct the whole problem. "In such cases, T3 therapy can often be used to predictably, effectively, reproducibly, and quickly influence the system to return to a normal pattern of function."[2]

When the metabolic "oven" is undercooking and the temperature gauge is stuck anywhere below 98.6, nasty things happen. Every function and every system of the body is affected. So much so that the person may feel like he or she is literally falling apart.

Such was the case with Trish Hazzard. Hers had been a high energy, on-the-go lifestyle. Not only was she employed full-time as a piano teacher, but she also found time to simultaneously maintain a 3.95 grade point average as a full-time college student, do aerobics three times a week, walk two miles every day at noon, produce various writing projects, do gourmet cooking, and cater her daughter's engagement party for eighty people. She called it being a "200 percent person," and that was the way she liked to live her life. At least, that was up until the accident.

The weather in her part of town looked just fine that morning in late April when she left home and headed for work. April snow storms, however, are not uncommon in Colorado Springs and can whip down the nearby mountains in a flash. On her way north up the interstate through town, she found herself smack dab in the middle of a doozie. Rain, sleet, hail, snow, slush—it was coming down fast and furious. She cautiously made her way along her usual route, but sometimes no matter how careful you are, you can find yourself reaping the consequences of somebody else's mistakes. On her way around a truck, it pulled into her lane. Swerving to avoid being hit, she skidded into a patch of ice, catapulted across several lanes of traffic, and rolled her jeep three times down an incline next to the road.

"I was lucky I wasn't killed," she recalls. But there have been times since when she wishes she had been. The pain she experienced as a result of the accident was excruciating. "My joints ached, my back ached, my neck ached, I had pinched nerves, I had TMJ, and the pains in my stomach were terrible."

Severe whiplash, according to her doctor, was the cause of her muscle and nerve pain. And although physical therapy seemed only to make things worse, it was all the medical community currently had to offer. So confident was her doctor in his diagnosis of her problem that no MRI was ever done, a test that would have revealed more than simple X-rays. Her constant complaints and protests that something else was wrong with her neck fell upon deaf ears. "They told me I didn't know what I was talking about, that it was whiplash and nothing more."

As for her abdominal problems, three exploratory surgeries were performed without success.

"I had so many things wrong with me. And each specialist I was seeing went to work on some isolated symptom, ignoring the big picture. I carried on that way for over a year, pushing myself to work, hurting all over but believing that nothing was really wrong with me because the doctors were telling me so. I just got worse, and worse, and worse. When I'd come home from work, I'd lie down on the couch for a ten-minute nap and wind up being "out" for the night. At one point I slept for fifty-two hours straight. For the first year, all I did outside of work was sleep. I was a real mess!"

After a year of living in the prison of excruciating pain, Trish decided that she didn't want to live anymore. "None of the doctors I'd been seeing was able to really help me. I was absolutely suicidal because of the constant pain and the lack of medical hope. I'd reached the end of my rope. The mental-health therapist I was seeing, Dr. Donna Underwood, made me promise to go see a local osteopathic physician named George Juetersonke."

Juetersonke is to medicine what Sherlock Holmes is to crime fighting, a super sleuth. He refers to his practice as "third-line medicine." First there are the general practitioners, then the specialists. If neither of them can figure out what's happening in the body, then come practitioners like him, "third liners."

"I went to see Dr. J, and he spent two hours with me going over everything, my entire medical history," recalls Trish. "He asked questions about every detail of the accident, and about every single symptom I'd been having since."

Well versed in the telltale signs of Wilson's syndrome, Dr. J had Trish take her temperature three times a day while she was active, for ten days. Although blood tests done by previous doctors had not detected a problem with low thyroid functioning, he said that body temperature was the only clear indicator. Sure enough, she was undercooking at 96 to 97 degrees—far from the 98.6 mark that our bodies are designed to function best at.

There had been structural damage to Trish's body due to the accident. In fact, later she discovered that she actually had three herniated disks in her neck that the doctor who had insisted on physical therapy had not detected.

"Had I tripped or fallen, I likely would have severed my spinal cord and been paralyzed from the neck down. The pain that had been dismissed so readily as simple whiplash was much more serious. I was right, after all."

But the structural damage did not account for the low body temperature. It was obvious that her body had gone into the conservation mode and never switched back to the productivity mode. The trauma of the accident had shut down her thyroid hormone system, and although her spirit was telling her to recapture her productive lifestyle of the past, her flesh was weak—"Leave me alone, I'm tired, I want to sleep." In fact, her body seemed to be slowly falling apart. T3 therapy was of vital importance to overall recovery.

"Within two doses I felt better. I felt better all over. Dramatic improvement! I was excited. I was really in tune with what was happening in my body. If anything was going to help me, I would notice it right away. And with T3, it was amazing!"

Along the way, the doctor also discovered that her adrenals were not secreting enough of yet another hormone called DHEA, a steroid the body naturally produces that aids the process of retarding and destroying cancer cells.

"T3 and DHEA have made me feel the best I've felt in the years since that accident," says a convinced Trish. "You should see the before and after pictures. Dr. J. has them. It's amazing! The day I came into his office I was all swollen up. You could tell I was full of poison and sickness. My eyes were all glassy, and there was this pallor on my skin. Just yuck! In the picture he took a year later, I don't even look like the same person. I'd lost weight, my color was good, and I looked healthy."

Dr. Juetersonke and the hormone supplements he prescribed have been helping to reset Trish's metabolic thermostat. She hasn't totally regained her old form, but she's headed in the right direction.

"Dr. J and T3 have saved my life! My husband will attest to that. If it wasn't for our doctor and his treatments, and his willingness to listen to me and believe me when I told him something wasn't right, I'd be dead today."

QUOTES

"What sets Wilson's Syndrome apart from many other uncomplicated problems is that it just so happens to affect one of the most fundamental regulating processes of the body. And because of this fact, it can affect essentially every other process in the body by affecting the body temperature. This significant point is what gives Wilson's Syndrome its extreme importance. It's like the one card on the bottom of a house of cards that can't be removed without the whole house collapsing."

—Dennis Wilson, M.D.
WILSON'S SYNDROME

"Here I was, a registered nurse with some record of success in helping others to get well, and I couldn't find a way to get help for myself. The morning 'ache all over feeling,' headaches, more and more pronounced fatigue and trouble focusing, lasted longer and longer each day. . . . The increasing signs that my body wasn't functioning well (increased infections, skin problems, neurological problems, mental problems) were evident. It seemed to me that something was terribly wrong with my metabolism, but no physician could find a test to substantiate that, and I was becoming depressed. . . . Still, I arrived at Wilson's Syndrome Treatment Center with a fair amount of

*skepticism. His explanation of WS made sense and his explana-
tion of its cause and the way it could be corrected sounded
promising. About everything he described I found to be true. I
was amazed to find my average body temperature was so much
below normal. I was likewise amazed when my troublesome
symptoms decreased as my average temperature increased. I
was so prepared not to believe what I heard that I couldn't
accept at first that I felt much better within a week after I
started the treatment plan."*

—Betty J., R.N.
WILSON'S SYNDROME

*"As I learn more about this disorder, I can recognize the begin-
ning of the symptoms 20 years earlier. At age 30, after having 4
children in 6¹/₂ years, relocating 5 times in 8 years, I was diagnosed by a rural doctor as having a mild thyroid condition. He
did not use blood tests, but took my oral temperature, blood
pressure, and checked knee jerk reflex. My blood pressure/tem-
perature were low and reflexes sluggish. At that time I was
placed on a small amount of thyroid. Even though I was about
10 to 15 pounds over normal weight, I quickly lost weight and
felt good. We relocated, however, in 12 months, and I was not
able to have the prescription renewed. Each MD after that
stated that I did not have a thyroid deficiency.*

*"In 1976, I had a total hysterectomy with a traumatic post
surgical wound infection. Within several weeks, I returned to my
high pressure job, but it seemed that I began to feel progressively
worse. Even though I was an excellent job performer, my heart
was no longer in my work. My weight began to increase 5 to 6
pounds per year; I noticed that my oral temperature was about 1
degree below normal. On visits to the physician, I would explain
my symptoms and state that I had previously taken thyroid. The
physician would complete an EKG and blood chemistry profile,
and tell me that I was very healthy. Once I even visited a psychologist who also informed me that except for mild depression
due to my job stress, I was very healthy even mentally.*

"Last fall was the first time I recognized that my symptoms

*were possibly related. I scheduled a visit with Dr. Wilson. I
could hardly believe it. It became so obvious. I have been
under treatment for 3-4 months. My body temperature is not
yet totally stabilized, but I feel like a new person. The joint
pains have completely disappeared. I started a 1,200 calorie
diet 5 weeks ago and I'm losing about 2¹/₂ pounds per week
with no difficulty. The fatigue and depression have been eliminated. My nails and hair are growing back. My nails are
stronger. The chest pains, indigestion/dyspepsia/flatus are
gone. My quality of life has improved 100%, and my husband
and I have even started playing golf and other recreational
activities together that we have not done in years. How I wish
that 20 years ago this had been diagnosed. Even 5 years ago
would have been a blessing."*

—Elizabeth W., R.N.
WILSON'S SYNDROME

FRAN HAMPTON
PMS

At forty-three, Fran Hampton is competing with kids half her
age as she argues her way through law school. The end of the recent
school year found her rated twelfth out of 112 in the class. Not bad
for someone who only a couple of years earlier couldn't muster
the physical strength and emotional willpower to get out of bed
and face her world.

"I was nearing forty then and going through a really bad period
of my life. It was the strangest thing. I wasn't getting any rest at
night. I just couldn't sleep. And I started going through really
depressed periods. I remember one time there was an important
banquet being held where my husband was to receive recognition for his work. I was in such bad shape that I couldn't get myself
up out of bed to go. I just can't put into words how miserable
I'd become."

Something was definitely amiss. Fran had always been a woman
of dreams and ambition, with the guts and gumption to make those
dreams and ambitions come true. For a number of years she'd been

a corporate controller and a CPA. Recently she and her husband had set their sights on completing master's degrees in computer resource management. Then in her very last class, she wondered if she had the wherewithal to finish.

"I was at my wits end. My body and my mind seemed to be falling apart. I felt so bad that I was considering just dropping the class and forgetting about the degree."

About that time, Fran made an appointment with a neural psychiatrist. Her oldest son had been under his care for a learning disorder. She thought perhaps he could run some tests and get to the bottom of what was happening to her.

"His initial conclusion seemed to point toward depression, so he put me on Prozac, an antidepressant. I got worse. I went back to see him—no, in fact, my husband went back to report to him how much worse I'd become. For days on end I wouldn't get out of bed. And I'd cry at the drop of a hat."

Following further tests, the antidepressant was discontinued. "I think you're having some sort of a nutritional problem," the psychiatrist said. "There's a doctor here in town that I think would be well worth your seeing. I'll even make the appointment for you. His name is George Juetersonke, and he's an osteopathic physician."

If you've already read Trish Hazzard's story, you know that Dr. Juetersonke enjoys getting to the root of a problem. Not only does he know his medicine, but he also knows his nutrition. If indeed Fran was suffering from a nutritional deficiency, Dr. J was the man to see.

"First he tapped the side of my face with one of those little hammers to check my reflexes there," recalls Fran. "My mouth just sort of slid all over my face. After a few additional tests and questions, he concluded that I very well may have a magnesium deficiency, perhaps even a profound deficiency."

Magnesium is a very important mineral to the human metabolic system. In addition to migraine headaches, other symptoms of deficiency can include muscle cramps, tension headaches, palpitations, asthma, insomnia, anxiety, vasospastic angina (chest pains), worsening of mitral valve prolapse, constipation, numbness, and tingling sensations.

"That certainly accounted for the problems I was having," recalls Fran. "I also realized that it was always worse from the middle of my menstrual cycle through the end of my period. Those two weeks were always terrible. I'd be a fairly normal human being again for the next two weeks, but then the whole thing would start all over again."

Magnesium shots were just what the doctor ordered, and Fran was taught how to give them to herself. She was also instructed to start taking a natural form of progesterone, made from wild yams. The body converts it into whatever kind of hormone is needed. It seemed clear that her mineral balance problems were related to monthly hormonal changes. It may even have had something to do with hormonal changes associated with the nearing of menopause (her problems began as she approached forty), although she's now forty-three and has yet to experience "the change."

"I was in such bad shape that day when I left Dr. J's office that I couldn't find the pharmacy to pick up what he had prescribed for me," Fran recalls. "I was crying and crying, and had to stop and call my husband to come help me. Talk about messed up and confused! But look at me now. I'm in the top 10 percent of my class in law school. That's quite an improvement!"

Improvement, indeed! Within weeks of beginning the program of magnesium supplements and progesterone, Fran was back on her feet and headed toward recovery of her old self again. Sleep returned to her nights, and clarity to her brain. Having regained her old vigor, she pursued a degree as a CFP (Certified Financial Planner) to add to her already achieved master's, then went on to law school.

"I don't know how I would have handled life apart from Dr. J getting me all straightened out," she admits. "We've since moved to Virginia from Colorado. When I told a doctor here the kinds of treatments Dr. J had done for me, he just laughed. He'd never heard of such a thing. I guess if all of this had happened to me after we'd moved, I'd probably still be on a psychiatrist's couch taking antidepressant drugs. When I explained how much better I'd gotten under Dr. J's care, the doctor said, 'Well, if he's done so much for you, maybe you just ought to keep him as your doctor.' That's exactly what I'm doing. I wouldn't dream of giving up contact with Dr. J. I thank God for him and for the psychiatrist who had the wisdom to point me in his direction."

FURTHER READING
CATARACTS
Nutrition, Health and Disease by Gary Price Todd, M.D. (Atlen, PA: Whitford Press, 1985).

What Your Doctor Won't Tell You by Jane Heimlich (New York: HarperPerennial, 1990), chapter 9, "Cataract Surgery—Another Unnecessary Operation?"

WILSON'S SYNDROME
Wilson's Syndrome by Dennis Wilson, M.D. (Orlando, FL; Cornerstone Publishing Co, 1991).

RESOURCE
For more information about Wilson's syndrome, or to order the book:

Wilson's Syndrome Foundation
P.O. Box 916206
Longwood, FL 32791-6206
(800)621-7006

NOTES
1. Dennis Wilson, M.D., *Wilson's Syndrome* (Orlando, FL: Cornerstone Publishing Co., 1991), page 40.
2. Wilson, page 36.

EPILOGUE

The magazine article told the story of Susan, a thirty-six-year-old woman who had watched as breast cancer struck her mother at forty-six, then killed her oldest sister at thirty-eight, and later took the lives of two cousins in their thirties. So when she learned that her remaining sister, at forty-one, had come down with the dread disease, she did what any rational person would do. She panicked.

"I knew I wanted to have my breasts off. I was so afraid I was going to get cancer before I could."

Her sister supported her in that decision, even though the benefits are unproven. "I felt like to save our family, all women had to get their breasts off. The feeling is, 'You can cut anything off. I just want to live.'"

The article went on to document current genetic research. Scientists are looking for the faulty genes in our bodies that are responsible for the development of various degenerative diseases. The implication behind this research is (1) that if someone has certain genetic predispositions toward a disease, its development is inevitable, and (2) that if those genes run in a person's family, perhaps he or she ought to consider removing the body part that is prone to degenerative weakness before it gets that way.

If breast cancer runs in your family, cut 'em off. And following that logic, if you have inherited a genetic predisposition toward colon cancer, get that sucker out of there right away. Start collecting your waste in a bag glued to your side. And brain tumors, oh my! Have them get that brain out of there, pronto, before it starts to give you trouble.

I have a sneaking suspicion that the medical researchers and doctors who promote and perform removal of body parts in the name of "preventive" medicine must have already had one of those brain jobs done themselves.

In another magazine, a different article tells the story of angry women banding together into activist groups. Their intention is to put pressure on Congress to direct more money toward breast cancer research. In fact, they plan to sponor races all over the country to raise money for such research projects. They hand over to various government-sponsored medical organizations all the money they collect, hoping that some day somebody will come up with medicines or genetic engineering that will erradicate cancer from our world.

They might just as well flush that money down the toilet!

Drugs don't cure, and DNA is not absolute destiny. Drugs may temporarily halt a disease process and mask symptoms, but they don't cure anything. And family history is not a concrete roadmap to your future. What a scientist may see in your genetic makeup is not necessarily an indication of what you'll experience in your health. Reports coming out of the Institute of Medicine (part of the National Academy of Sciences) conclude that genetic tests are seldom perfect predictors of health risk.

The real culprits behind most of our degenerative diseases today, particularly the biggest killers, are diet and lifestyle choices. We don't need to sponsor more research into finding miracle cures. What we need is to make better choices about what we're feeding ourselves. We live in a world where it's not what's in our genes that counts, but what's in our mouths.

Our hope is that the stories you have read in this book have helped to convince you and teach you about making better choices about what you put into your body.

RESOURCES

HealthQuarterly
The goals of this newletter are (1) to educate readers about nutrition, (2) to tell the stories of people who have used nutrition to win back their health, (3) to link readers with professionals who can help them, and (4) tell news about *Health*Quarters activities: A subscription is $15/year, and it's published quarterly.

Heath Resources
This is a list (currently forty-nine pages and growing) of health-care professionals who use nutrition to help others. We've compiled this list of practitioners from around the U.S. (M.D.'s, nutritionists, D.O.'s, chiropractors, etc.) who use nutrition and/or related nontoxic therapies in their practices. For a tax deductible donation of twenty-five dollars to *Health*Quarters we'll gladly send you the current copy of this list. The "hard cost" to *Health*Quarters for production and mailing is five dollars. All additional funds realized go to support our work. Make checks out to *Health*Quarters, and mail with your request to this address:

*Health*Quarters
6873 Prince Drive
Colorado Springs, CO 80918

A Cancer Battle Plan and *Healthy Habits*
These are two previous books we have written. *A Cancer Battle Plan* is the story of Anne's recovery from "terminal" cancer. *Healthy Habits* carries the subtitle *20 Simple Ways to Improve Your Health*. They are available at or through most major bookstores, health food stores, or religious bookstores. In the U.S. you can request a catalog and order them directly from the publisher, Piñon Press, at (800)366-7788, or in Canada from R. G. Mitchell Family Books at (416)499-4615.

OTHER NEWSLETTERS
There are many other nutrition-related newsletters available. We especially like these.

Back to the Garden
Health News from Hallelujah Acres (Subscription fee: free)
We like this one because it always includes within its sixteen pages several interviews with people who have used nutrition to win back their health over serious illness. Write or call:

> Hallelujah Acres
> P.O. Box 10
> Eidson, TN 37737
> (615)272-1800

Health and Healing
Tomorrow's Medicine Today (Subscription fee: $69/year)
This newsletter's author, Julian Whitaker, M.D., is a leading spokesman today for nutrition and other alternative forms of health care. We like his eight-page newsletter because it gives in-depth coverage to a few practical health topics each issue. Also, Dr. Whitaker keeps the reader well informed about the political side of medicine and how it impacts our freedom of choice. Write or call:

> Dr. Julian Whitaker's Health and Healing
> 7811 Montrose Road

Potomac, MD 20854
(301)424-3700

Lifestyle for Health Newsletter (Subscription fee: $20/year)
Author Cheryl Townsley does a superb job of packing this
twelve-page newsletter with practical menu ideas, plus health
tips from the experts. If you want help in preparing healthy
meals, this is your newsletter. Ms. Townsley has also written
three nutrition-oriented cookbooks, which are available from
the address below, plus she has a fourth book called *Food
Smart! Eat Your Way to Better Health* (Piñon Press, 1994). One
complimentary issue is available with an SASE (legal size).
Write or call:

Lifestyle for Health
P.O. Box 3871
Littleton, CO 80161
(303)771-9357

The Nutrition Reporter (Subscription fee: $24)
Eight pages packed with the latest findings from studies on
nutrition, plus interviews with professionals who use nutritional
therapies in their practice. Write:

The Nutrition Reporter
P.O. Box 5505
Aloha, OR 97006-5505

*Townsend Letter for Doctors: An Informal Letter Magazine for
Doctors Communicating with Doctors (Subscription fee:
$69/month)*
Extremely informative and educational! Each issue is 100-plus
pages packed with findings and opinions from the health-care
community on a wide range of alternative health-care issues
and practices. Reviews of new books, plus comments on latest
happenings within the world of medical politics are also

included. Some articles border on the "too technical for the layperson" side of things, but if you're serious about becoming a student of the world of health care, and in particular health care with an "alternative" slant, add this newsletter to your "must read" list. Write or call:

Townsend Letter for Doctors
911 Tyler Street
Port Townsend, WA 98368-6541
(206)385-6021

MAGAZINES

The number of well-written and informative magazines concerning nutrition and related health issues is growing every month. Here are a few that we like.

Delicious (Your Magazine of Natural Health) (Subscription fee: $20/U.S., $24/Canada)

New Hope Communications, Inc.
1301 Spruce Street
Boulder, CO 80302
(303)939-8840

Let's Live (America's Foremost Health and Preventive Magazine)

Let's Live Magazine
P.O. Box 74908
Los Angeles, CA 90004
(800)676-4333

Natural Health (The Guide to Well-Being) (Subscription fee: $24/U.S., $27/Canada)

Natural Health Magazine
P.O. Box 57320

Boulder, CO 80322-7320
(303)447-9330

*Vegetarian Times (Subscription fee: $23.95/U.S.,
$28.95/Canada)*

Vegetarian Times
P.O. Box 570
Oak Park, IL 60303
(800)435-9610

GLOSSARY

CHELATION THERAPY: Chelation comes from the Greek word *chele*, which means "claw." A synthetic amino acid called EDTA (ethylene diamine tetraacetic acid) is slowly dripped into a vein and, once in the bloodstream, claws or grasps heavy toxic metals in the body, allowing them to be removed from the system. This use of chelation—to remove toxic metals such as lead or mercury—was approved by the FDA in the early 1950s. Chelation has another effect, which is to restore circulation to arteries blocked by plaque. (*Source:* Jane Heimlich)

CLINICAL ECOLOGY AND CLINICAL ECOLOGISTS: A deeper realm of allergy and immunology fascinated many physicians since the mid-1970s. This is now incorporated into the field of clinical ecology. It involves human interaction with the environment and its effect on human health and disease.

Clinical ecologists are physicians who evaluate and treat chronic illness on the basis of allergy, immune response (and immune weakness), and nutrition. Therapy may involve isolation from allergens, dietary changes, and an "orthomolecular" approach to nutritional supplements—that is, using greater amounts of various nutrients to support the body's functions and to alter abnormal physiology and correct functional or metabolic nutritional imbalances. (*Source:* Elson M. Haas, M.D.)

HOMEOPATHY: The basis of this kind of health-care treatment is that "like cures like." Subjecting the body to very diluted amounts of an antigen (a toxin, foreign protein, bacteria, etc.)

234

triggers a protective reaction within the immune system. In other words, the body is exposed to such a small dosage of the antigen that it can't actually cause the disease, but enough that the immune system can build up a natural tolerance to it.

MUSCLE RESPONSE TESTING: A technique for determining food allergies. Also referred to as Applied Kinesiology. The concept behind MRT is that our bodies, just like all other matter, generate an electrical current. Scientists and doctors have recognized this for years. Foods to which an individual is allergic will disrupt the flow of this electrical current, thus making muscles weak.

The testing is conducted by having the patient stand with his or her strongest arm outstretched from the body at a 90 degree angle, palm down. In the other hand, the person holds a food item (non-processed) against his stomach. While his mouth is shut and his feet are flat on the floor, the person conducting the test stands in front of him and presses down on his outstretched arm at the wrist.

A strong muscle feels as though it locks when tested. This indicates that the electrical current has not been disrupted. No allergy. On the other hand, a weak muscle gives way when tested. Whatever is being held to the stomach can cause an allergic reaction in the body.

For more detailed information refer to *Your Body Doesn't Lie* (Warner Books) by John Diamond, M.D.

NATUROPATHY AND NATUROPATHIC DOCTORS: Naturopathic doctors are the only primary-care physicians clinically trained in a wide variety of medical systems. Their education is built upon conventional medical sciences, but the treatments they learn to administer for illness and disease are significantly different from those taught in a conventional medical school or employed by a typical M.D. (medical doctor). In other words, they have studied the same questions as an M.D., but their answers are different.

Naturopathic medicine is the philosophy and practice of treating disease by following the principles and laws of nature, rather than utilizing chemicals, drugs, surgery, or other artificial or intrusive methods. Naturopaths endeavor to stimulate the body's innate healing resources through employment of a variety of methods, some of which include therapeutic nutrition, homeopathic medicine, herbs and botanical medicine, massage and naturopathic manipulative therapy, acupuncture, and acupressure.

The degree of Doctor of Naturopathic Medicine (N.D.) requires four years of graduate level study at a naturopathic medical college. The admissions requirements for these schools are comparable to those of conventional medical schools. There are currently three such colleges in the U.S.:

Bastyr College
144 NE 54th Street
Seattle, WA 98105
(206)523-9585

National College
11231 SE Market Street
Portland, OR 97216
(503)255-4860

Southwest College
6535 East Osborn Road
Scottsdale, AZ 85251
(602)990-7424

As a distinct American health-care profession, naturopathic medicine will soon be 100 years old. In the early 1900s, practitioners of various medical disciplines brought together what they knew of natural healing methods and formed the first professional naturopathic medical societies. By the 1920s naturopathic medical conventions drew more that 10,000 practitioners from around the country. At that point, twenty different colleges of naturopathic medicine were in operation.

In the '40s and '50s, naturopathic medicine experienced a

decline in numbers of participating doctors. It was a time when pharmaceutical drugs and emerging medical technologies seemed to promise the future elimination of all disease. It was also a time when the American Medical Association (AMA) used its political muscle to strictly limit the practice of naturopathy in the United States.

Over the last several decades, however, there has been a growing resurgence of interest in naturopathic medicine, as the health-conscious consumer in this country began to seek out alternatives to conventional medicine.

OSTEOPATHY AND OSTEOPATHIC PHYSICIANS: Osteopathic physicians (D.O.) and medical doctors (M.D.) receive the same basic training and both are licensed by the American Medical Association (AMA). To the average layperson, D.O. and M.D. are basically interchangeable—both considered "medical doctors." Osteopathy, however, incorporates a broader view of illness and health, blending together drug therapies with a hands-on manipulation technique similar to that found in chiropractic. An osteopath, in other words, has more tools in his medical kit than does an M.D. Through musculoskeletal manipulation, an osteopath can stimulate the body toward certain self-healing processes. A D.O. prescribes drugs far less frequently than an M.D. Osteopaths tend to be more open-minded about other forms of therapy, as well—many are getting the necessary training to add these to their own practices (herbology, acupuncture, nutrition, chelation therapy, etc.).

AUTHORS

They've been called "health nuts" and "food freaks." Dave and Anne Frähm, however, prefer to think of themselves as just average folk helping other average folk learn how to take better care of their bodies through what they put into their mouths. It was, after all, what Anne eventually learned about nutrition that helped her turn the tide against her own case of so-called "terminal" breast cancer.

They make a good team, the Frähm's. Dave researches and writes. Anne researches and speaks. Her audience stretches from sea to shining sea (and then some) and has included church and civic groups, radio and television audiences, gatherings of alternative health-care providers, and nutrition support groups. Their previous books are *A Cancer Battle Plan* (Piñon Press, 1992) and *Healthy Habits* (Piñon Press, 1993). Dave has also written *The Great Niche Hunt*, which is now out of print.

Together they give direction to an organization they began in 1991 called *Health*Quarters, a donor-supported education and resource center for better health through nutrition. For more information about *Health*Quarters write or call: *Health*Quarters, 6873 Prince Drive, Colorado Springs, CO 80918; (719)593-8694.

There are two "up and coming" Frähms from this clan. Jessica, currently a teenager, has inherited her father's love of a good argument and looks to make a great lawyer. Ben, also a teen, has inherited his mother's gifts as an artist and mechanic.

MORE GREAT IDEAS FOR A HEALTHIER LIFESTYLE!

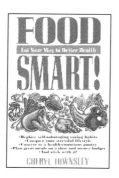

More and more Americans want to develop a healthier diet and lifestyle. But many are too busy or just don't have enough good information to make the kinds of changes they want to make. With *Food Smart!* you'll learn how to: ▸replace your self-sabotaging eating habits ▸conquer your stressful lifestyle ▸convert to a health-conscious pantry ▸plan great meals without spending a lot of time or money ▸and more!
Food Smart! (# 0891098399) $12

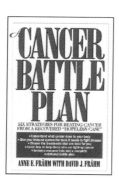

In *A Cancer Battle Plan*, former "hopeless case" cancer patient Anne Frähm shares the strategies she used to beat terminal cancer in just five weeks. Backed by the research of more than 30 doctors, nutritionists, and cancer scientists, this book also includes menus, recommended resources, and plenty of practical tips on how to transition into a healthier lifestyle.
A Cancer Battle Plan (# 0891096906) $12

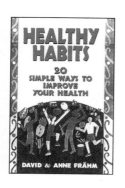

Studies show that more than half of all diseases are related to nutrition and lifestyle and are thus preventable. In *Healthy Habits*, the Frähms present the best and most "do-able" advice from a broad cross-section of nutrition, health, and wellness experts. Topics include: ▸what to do with meat and dairy products ▸how to deal with guests, dinner invitations, and restaurant meals ▸the best forms of exercise ▸handling stress ▸and more.
Healthy Habits (# 0891097546) $12

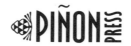